CLEAR ALIGNERS REVOLUTIONIZING ORTHODONTICSS

Dr. Pramod Kumar

Senior Resident

JLNMCH Bhagalpur

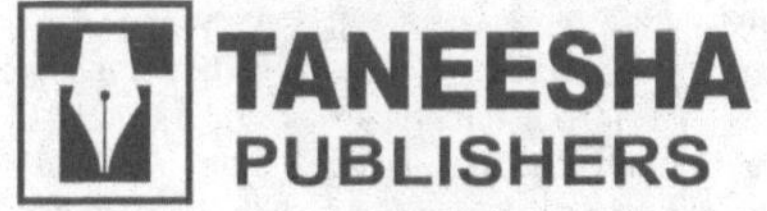

Title   : Clear Aligners Revolutionizing Orthodontics

Author   : Dr. Pramod Kumar

Edition   : First (October, 2024)

ISBN   : 9789348037053

Published by

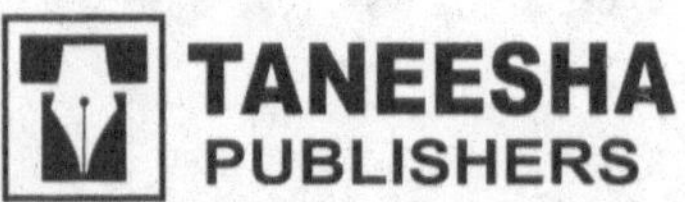 **TANEESHA PUBLISHERS** | *A Venture by -* **PRACHI DIGITAL PUBLICATION**

Regd. Add.: 254, Khuriyakhatta No. 10, Bindukhatta,
Lalkuan, Nainital - 262402, Uttarakhand, India
Website : www.taneeshapublishers.in
E-mail : taneeshapublishers@gmail.com
Phone : +91 845481 2712, +91 976041 7980

Printed by :

Manipal Technologies Limited, Bengaluru - 560001, Karnataka

Acknowledgement

This book would not have been possible without the support and guidance of several individuals and organizations who contributed their knowledge, expertise, and encouragement throughout the writing process.

First and foremost, I would like to express my heartfelt gratitude to all the dental professionals and orthodontists who shared their insights and experiences with me. Your wealth of knowledge and practical advice enriched this book immensely.

A special thanks to the patients who allowed their cases to be shared as part of this work. Your stories and testimonials provide invaluable real-world perspectives that give life to the concepts discussed within these pages.

I also extend my deepest appreciation to the pioneers and innovators in the field of clear aligner technology, whose relentless pursuit of excellence continues to drive this industry forward. Your dedication to transforming orthodontic care inspired many of the ideas explored here.

I am sincerely grateful to my family and friends for their unwavering support, patience, and encouragement throughout this project. Your belief in my work kept me motivated every step of the way.

To my editor and publishing team, thank you for your guidance and for bringing clarity and polish to this book. Your expertise and attention to detail were instrumental in shaping the final product.

Lastly, to all readers and dental professionals who choose to engage with this book, thank you for your interest. I hope this work serves as a valuable resource and enhances your understanding of the evolving world of clear aligner orthodontics.

A million words cannot express the strength of gratitude that I feel towards my wife **Mrs Madhuri Kumari** and my daughters **Maya Vasu** and **Mona Suhasi** for their humble prayer and unconditional love. Their blessings made this endeavour successful. The support, understanding, love and unflinching encouragement from my mother **Mrs. Tarini Devi** my uncle **Sri Vidya Sagar** have given me the impetus to carry on. The cooperation of my family in terms of patience, perseverance, and faith in me kept me motivated and encouraged me to work harder. I would like to remember my father Late Krishna Sagar for his blessings. **Last, but not the least, I express my gratitude to all, who directly or indirectly provided their esteemed cooperation that made me complete this dissertation.**

- **Dr. Pramod Kumar**

Abstract

Title: Clear Aligners: Revolutionizing Orthodontics

Clear aligners represent a significant advancement in orthodontic treatment, offering a modern, aesthetic alternative to traditional metal braces. This book delves into the multifaceted world of clear aligners, exploring their development, technology, and application in contemporary orthodontics.

Chapter 1: Introduction to Clear Aligners sets the stage by tracing the history of orthodontic treatments and the evolution from metal braces to the emergence of clear aligners. It provides an overview of the technology behind aligners and the rationale for their use in correcting malocclusions.

Chapter 2: How Clear Aligners Work examines the underlying science and mechanics of clear aligners, including the materials used, the treatment process, and the role of 3D scanning and digital modeling in creating personalized treatment plans.

Chapter 3: Types of Clear Aligners offers a detailed comparison of major clear aligner brands such as Invisalign, ClearCorrect, and Smile Direct Club. It also contrasts in-office aligners with direct-to-consumer options and assesses their suitability for various dental corrections.

Chapter 4: Advantages of Clear Aligners highlights the key benefits of clear aligners, including their aesthetic appeal, comfort, and ease of maintenance. It also discusses the predictability of treatment outcomes through digital planning.

Chapter 5: Limitations and Challenges addresses the potential drawbacks of clear aligners, including their limitations for complex cases, cost considerations, patient compliance, and possible discomfort.

Chapter 6: Patient Experience and Journey details the typical patient journey from initial consultation through treatment and retention. It covers the importance of adherence to treatment protocols and the management of common issues like discomfort and oral hygiene.

Chapter 7: Clinical Applications and Case Studies presents real-world applications of clear aligners through case studies, illustrating their effectiveness in treating various orthodontic problems. This chapter includes before-and-after results, the role of orthodontists, and patient testimonials.

Chapter 8: Technological Innovations in Clear Aligners explores recent advancements in aligner technology, including 3D printing, AI in treatment planning, and the future of teledentistry. It discusses how these innovations enhance treatment customization and patient experience.

Chapter 9: Clear Aligners vs. Traditional Braces provides a comprehensive comparison between clear aligners and traditional braces, considering effectiveness, cost, patient satisfaction, and lifestyle impacts. It also examines the ideal patient profiles for each option.

Chapter 10: The Business of Clear Aligners analyzes the growing market for clear aligners, including industry trends, marketing strategies, and regulatory considerations. It also explores the roles of general dentists and orthodontists in providing aligner therapy.

Chapter 11: The Future of Clear Aligners looks ahead to emerging technologies and trends in the field of clear aligners, including new brands, advancements in orthodontic care, and potential improvements in patient outcomes.

The Conclusion summarizes the book's key points and reflects on the ongoing evolution of clear aligners, emphasizing their increasing popularity and acceptance in mainstream orthodontics. The Appendix provides a glossary of key terms, answers to frequently asked questions, and additional resources for both patients and professionals.

This book serves as a comprehensive guide for anyone interested in clear aligners, from prospective patients and dental professionals to industry stakeholders and researchers.

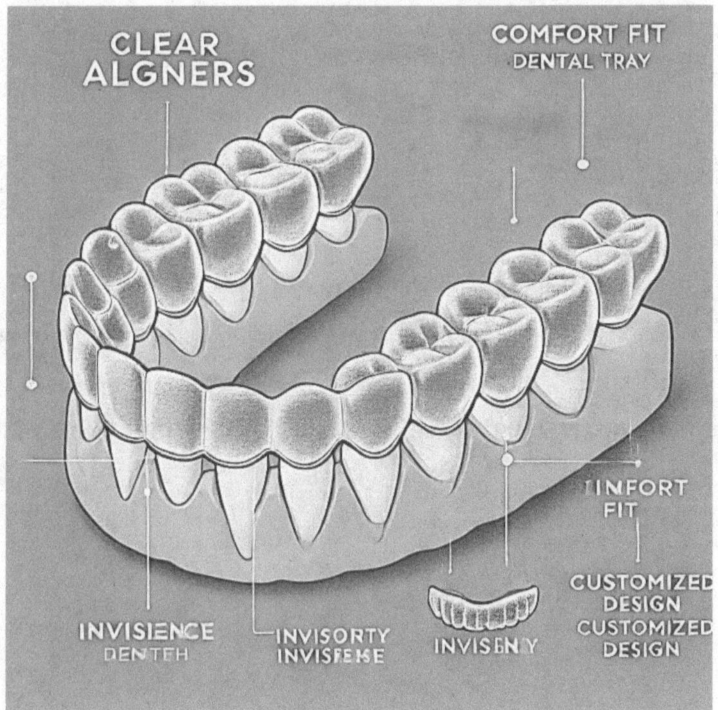

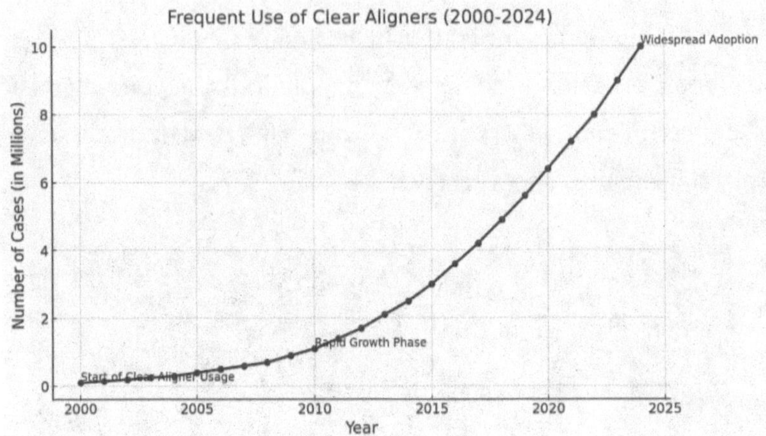

Line diagram illustrating the increasing use of clear aligners from the year 2000 to 2024. The plot shows a steady rise in usage over time, highlighting key milestones like the initial introduction and subsequent rapid growth, leading to widespread adoption by 2024.

Chapter 1

Introduction to Clear Aligners History of Orthodontic Treatments

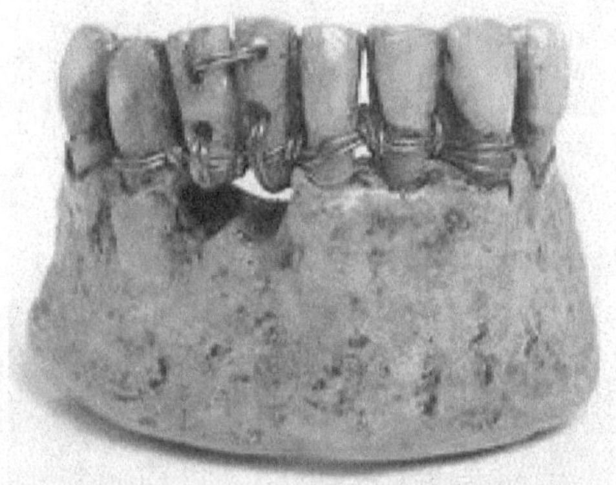

Orthodontics, the branch of dentistry focused on correcting irregularities of the teeth and jaws, has a rich and fascinating history. The desire to achieve straight teeth and a proper bite dates back thousands of years. Archaeological evidence from ancient Egypt suggests that rudimentary methods for aligning teeth were employed using metal bands and catgut, a type of natural fiber made from animal intestines. Similarly, ancient Greek and Roman civilizations used crude devices to push and pull misaligned teeth into better positions.

Fast forward to the 18th and 19th centuries, significant advancements began to take shape. The term "orthodontia" was coined by French dentist Pierre Fauchard, widely regarded as the father of modern dentistry. He developed the first modern orthodontic appliance, a horseshoe-shaped device designed to expand the dental arch. This period saw the use of early braces made from precious metals like gold and silver, which were custom-fitted to the patient's teeth. In the 20th century, the introduction of stainless steel revolutionized orthodontics. With the development of more sophisticated appliances, including fixed metal braces and various types of wires, orthodontic treatments became more effective and accessible. By the mid-20th century, innovations like elastic bands, headgear, and brackets further refined the practice, leading to the conventional metal braces still widely recognized today.

Emergence of Clear Aligners: From Metal Braces to Invisible Solutions

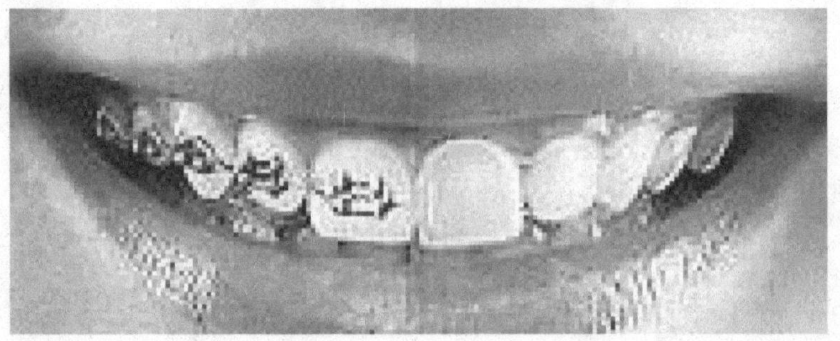

The shift from conspicuous metal braces to nearly invisible aligners represents a milestone in orthodontics. In the late 1990s, clear aligners emerged as a novel solution, offering patients a discreet, comfortable alternative to traditional braces. Align Technology, founded by Zia Chishti and Kelsey Wirth, pioneered this shift with the introduction of Invisalign in 1997. Utilizing 3D imaging, digital planning, and computer-aided manufacturing, the Invisalign system introduced a series of transparent plastic trays that gradually reposition teeth.

The development of clear aligners marked a significant breakthrough in both technology and patient experience. Unlike traditional braces that relied on metal brackets and wires to exert force on teeth, clear aligners use a sequence of custom-made trays that gently guide teeth into place. The idea of removable, nearly invisible orthodontic appliances was revolutionary, especially for adults and teenagers who were conscious of aesthetics.

Over the years, other companies like ClearCorrect, Smile Direct Club, and various smaller brands have joined the market, contributing to advancements in clear aligner technology. These companies have expanded treatment options and accessibility, making clear aligners a popular choice for mild to moderate malocclusions.

Overview of Clear Aligner Technology

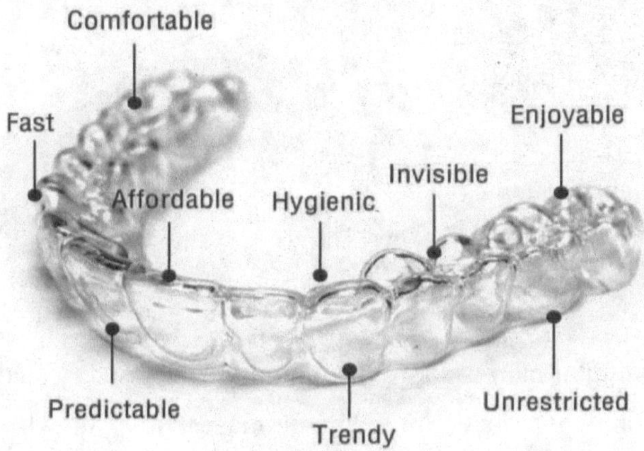

The effectiveness of clear aligners lies in the sophisticated blend of biomechanics, digital planning, and precise manufacturing. Clear aligners are made from advanced thermoplastic materials, which are both durable and flexible, designed to apply consistent, gentle pressure on teeth. The aligners are custom-fitted to each patient's dental anatomy, ensuring a snug fit that promotes movement over time.

The treatment process begins with a thorough assessment by an orthodontist or dentist. Using 3D scanners, a detailed digital impression of the patient's teeth is captured, replacing the need for traditional messy molds. The scanned images are then used to create a digital model, allowing the orthodontist to visualize the treatment from start to finish. This model serves as the foundation for designing a personalized treatment plan that predicts the movement of teeth at each stage.

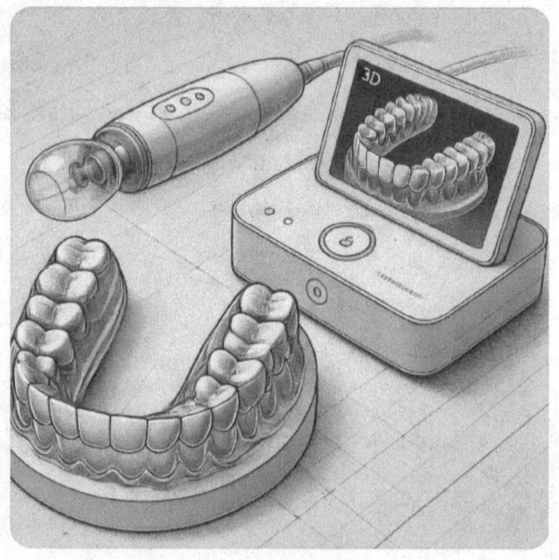

Once the digital plan is approved, the aligners are fabricated using 3D printing technology. The entire treatment may involve anywhere from 20 to 40 sets of aligners, depending on the complexity of the case. Each aligner is worn for approximately one to two weeks before progressing to the next one in the sequence, gradually shifting the teeth closer to the desired final position.

Understanding Malocclusions and the Need for Treatment

Malocclusions, or misalignments of the teeth and jaws, are one of the most common reasons for seeking orthodontic treatment. They can vary from minor spacing issues to severe bite problems that affect both function and appearance. Common types of malocclusions include crowding, spacing, overbite, underbite, crossbite, and open bite. Left untreated, these issues can lead to more serious problems, including difficulty chewing, speech impediments, jaw pain, and even periodontal disease.

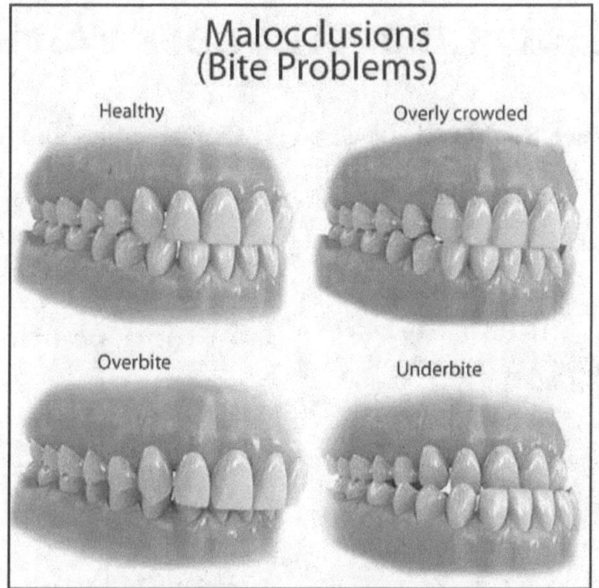

The need for orthodontic treatment extends beyond aesthetics. While many people pursue clear aligners for cosmetic reasons, correcting malocclusions has significant functional benefits. Proper alignment helps improve oral hygiene by reducing areas where plaque and food particles can accumulate. Additionally, a well-aligned bite ensures that forces are evenly distributed across the teeth during chewing, reducing the risk of tooth wear and temporomandibular joint (TMJ) disorders.

Clear aligners have proven to be an effective solution for a wide range of orthodontic issues, especially for mild to moderate cases. However, severe malocclusions, such as significant skeletal discrepancies or extreme crowding, may still require traditional braces or even surgical intervention. Despite these limitations, the versatility and convenience of clear aligners have made them a popular choice for millions of patients worldwide.

Chapter 2

How Clear Aligners Work

The Science Behind Clear Aligners: Biomechanics and Materials

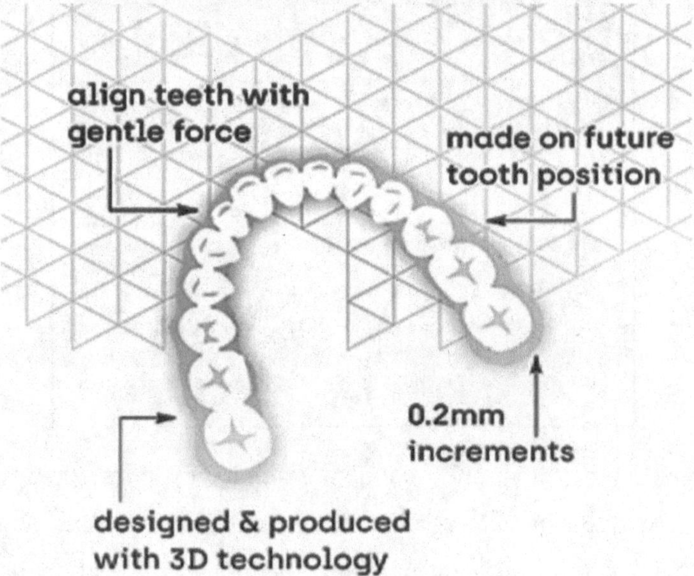

Clear aligners rely on a precise understanding of biomechanics and material science to achieve predictable and effective tooth movement. Unlike traditional braces that use wires and brackets, clear aligners apply gentle, controlled forces through a series of plastic trays. The aligners are made from advanced thermoplastic materials, such as medical-grade polyurethane resins. These materials are not only transparent and comfortable but also flexible enough to fit snugly over the teeth while being rigid enough to guide teeth gradually.

The science behind clear aligners lies in incremental tooth movement. Each aligner in the series is slightly different from the one before, exerting pressure on specific teeth to move them in the intended direction. The forces applied are carefully calculated to ensure that they are within safe biological limits, minimizing discomfort while allowing for effective bone remodeling and tooth movement.

Orthodontists use digital modeling software to plan the sequence of movements, determining the optimal path to align the teeth. By shifting the teeth in small, controlled increments (typically 0.25 mm to 0.33 mm per aligner), the treatment is both effective and comfortable for the patient.

Step-by-Step Process: From Consultation to Final Results

The clear aligner treatment journey can be broken down into several key stages:

1. **Initial Consultation and Assessment**: The process begins with a comprehensive evaluation by an orthodontist or dentist. During this consultation, the doctor assesses the patient's dental condition, examines bite alignment, and discusses treatment goals. If clear aligners are deemed suitable, the next step involves creating a detailed plan.

2. **3D Scanning and Digital Impressions**: Instead of traditional putty molds, modern clear aligner treatments use advanced 3D scanning technology to create digital impressions of the teeth. Scanners capture high-resolution images of the teeth, which are then used to generate a digital model. This digital model serves as the foundation for designing the treatment plan.

3. **Treatment Planning and Simulation**: Using specialized software, the orthodontist creates a virtual model that simulates the entire treatment process. This model shows the expected movement of teeth at each stage and gives the patient a preview of the final results. Once the plan is finalized and approved, it is sent for aligner production.

4. **Manufacturing of Aligners**: The aligners are fabricated using 3D printing technology. Each aligner is custom-made to fit the patient's teeth at specific stages of the treatment. Depending on the complexity of the case, the treatment may involve 20 to 40 sets of aligners.

5. **Wearing the Aligners**: Patients typically wear each set of aligners for 1 to 2 weeks, as instructed by their orthodontist. The aligners must be worn for 20 to 22 hours per day to achieve optimal results. Every new aligner in the series makes small adjustments to the teeth, gradually moving them closer to the desired final position.

6. **Monitoring and Adjustments**: Regular check-ups with the orthodontist ensure that the treatment is progressing as planned. Any necessary adjustments can be made along the way. Some treatments may involve the use of attachments—small tooth-colored bumps attached to certain teeth to enhance movement—or elastics to address specific bite issues.

7. **Completion and Retention**: Once the treatment is complete and the teeth have reached their final position, retainers are provided to maintain the results. Retainers are crucial to prevent teeth from shifting back to their original positions.

3D Scanning, Digital Modeling, and Treatment Planning

One of the key innovations in clear aligner therapy is the use of 3D scanning and digital modeling. Traditional orthodontics required physical impressions using putty, which could be uncomfortable and inaccurate. Modern clear aligner treatments use intraoral scanners that capture highly accurate digital impressions. The data from these scans are used to create a 3D model of the teeth and surrounding structures.

With the 3D model, the orthodontist uses specialized software to plan the treatment in detail. This digital treatment plan allows for precise control over each stage of tooth movement. The software can simulate the movement of individual teeth and show a step-by-step progression from start to finish. This predictive capability allows patients to see what their final smile will look like before the treatment even begins.

Aligners Manufacturing Process

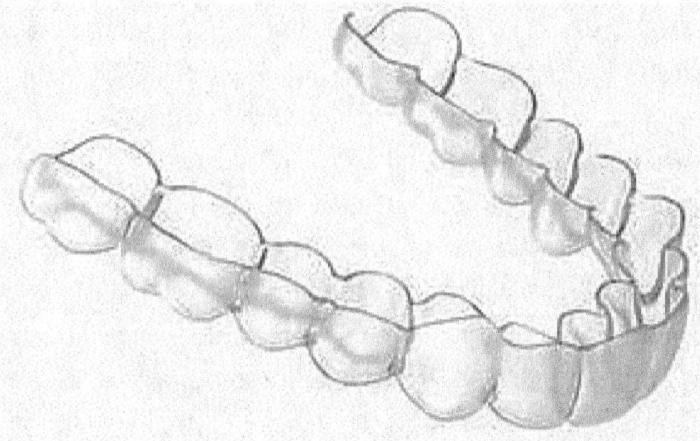

The manufacturing process for clear aligners is highly precise and automated, thanks to advancements in 3D printing and thermoplastic technology. Once the treatment plan is finalized, the digital models of each aligner are created. These models are then 3D printed to create molds, which are used to thermoform the aligners from sheets of transparent thermoplastic.

The aligners are trimmed and polished to ensure a comfortable fit and smooth edges. Each aligner is then labeled and packaged according to the sequence of use. The aligners are delivered to the orthodontist, who provides them to the patient with instructions on how and when to wear them.

Table 1- table summarizing the key stages in the clear aligner treatment process:

Stage	Description
1. Initial Consultation	Comprehensive evaluation by an orthodontist or dentist to assess dental condition and suitability for clear aligners. Treatment goals are discussed.
2. 3D Scanning and Impressions	High-resolution 3D scanning technology captures digital impressions of the teeth, replacing traditional putty molds.
3. Treatment Planning	Specialized software creates a digital model and simulates the treatment process. The patient can preview the final results before treatment begins.
4. Manufacturing of Aligners	Aligners are custom-made using 3D printing and thermoplastic molding processes. Each aligner corresponds to a specific stage in the treatment.
5. Wearing the Aligners	Patients wear each set of aligners for 1-2 weeks, typically 20-22 hours per day. Aligners gradually move teeth closer to the desired position.
6. Monitoring and Adjustments	Regular check-ups ensure the treatment is on track. Adjustments or additional aligners may be needed to optimize results.
7. Completion and Retention	After the final aligner is used, retainers are provided to maintain the new position of the teeth and prevent relapse.

Chapter 3

Types of Clear Aligners

Clear aligners have grown in popularity, and several brands offer different products to cater to varying orthodontic needs. Below is a comparison table that highlights the key features of major clear aligner brands, along with a detailed write-up discussing their differences, technologies, and suitability for specific cases.

Comparison Table: Major Clear Aligner Brands

Feature	Invisalign	Clear Correct	Smile Direct Club	Other Brands
Treatment Approach	In-office, supervised by a certified orthodontist or dentist	In-office, supervised by a certified provider	Direct-to-consumer (remote supervision by dental professionals)	Mixed approaches: some offer in-office care, others direct-to-consumer
Technology Used	Advanced 3D scanning, digital modeling, and SmartTrack ™ material	3D printing, digital modeling, ClearQuartz ™ material	At-home impression kit, digital planning, and regular remote check-ins	Varies by brand; some use AI-driven modeling and premium materials
Suitability for Complex Cases	Excellent for mild to complex cases (e.g., severe crowding,	Suitable for mild to moderate cases; can handle some complex	Primarily designed for mild cases (e.g., minor crowding, spacing)	Typically suited for mild to moderate cases

		cases		
	bite issues)	cases		
Cost	High (usually $3,000 to $8,000 depending on case complexity)	Moderate (usually $2,000 to $5,000)	Affordable (usually $1,500 to $2,500)	Varies by brand and service model
Customizatio n and Comfort	Highly customizable; uses proprietary materials for comfort and efficient movement	Customizable; flexible material designed for durability	Standard aligners; limited customization; designed for basic corrections	Varies; some offer customizatio n based on treatment needs
Duration of Treatment	6 months to 2 years depending on severity	6 months to 2 years	4 to 12 months	Varies based on brand and complexity
Supervision Level	High; regular in-person visits with an orthodontist or dentist	Moderate; in-office supervision by provider	Low; remote monitoring with periodic virtual check-ins	Varies; may involve virtual check-ins or in-office visits
Retainer Costs	Retainer included or available at additional cost	Retainer available at additional cost	Retainer included in most plans	Varies; usually an additional purchase

Invisalign

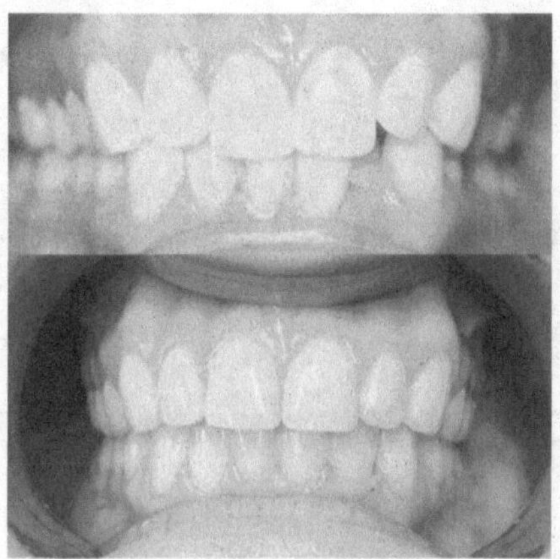

Invisalign is the market leader and one of the most established brands in clear aligner technology. It is widely known for its versatility, being suitable for treating mild to complex orthodontic cases. The company uses proprietary SmartTrack™ material, which provides comfort while delivering consistent pressure to move teeth efficiently. The treatment is fully supervised by certified orthodontists or dentists, who guide patients through regular in-person visits. The technology behind Invisalign includes advanced 3D scanning, AI-driven digital modeling, and precise treatment planning, making it highly effective for a range of dental corrections.

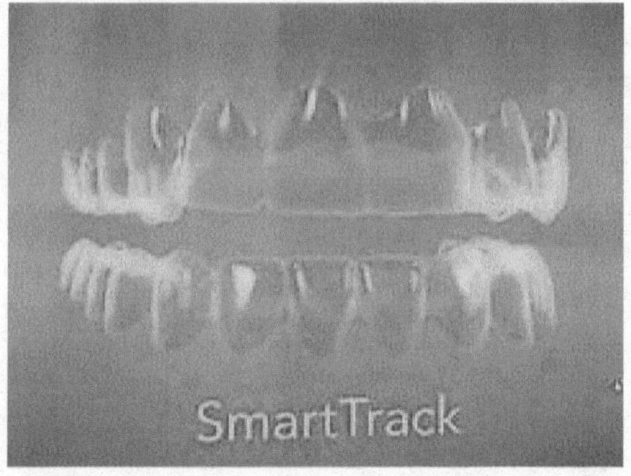

ClearCorrect

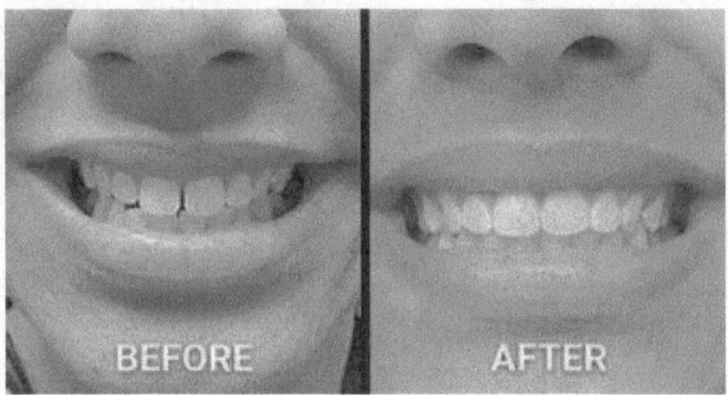

ClearCorrect is another popular option that offers both flexibility and affordability. Similar to Invisalign, it is administered by dental professionals who provide in-office consultations and supervision. ClearCorrect uses ClearQuartz™ material, designed to be durable and resistant to wear. It's often a preferred choice for those looking for an in-office aligner solution at a slightly lower cost compared to Invisalign. However, while it is effective for mild to moderate cases, it may not be as comprehensive as Invisalign for complex malocclusions.

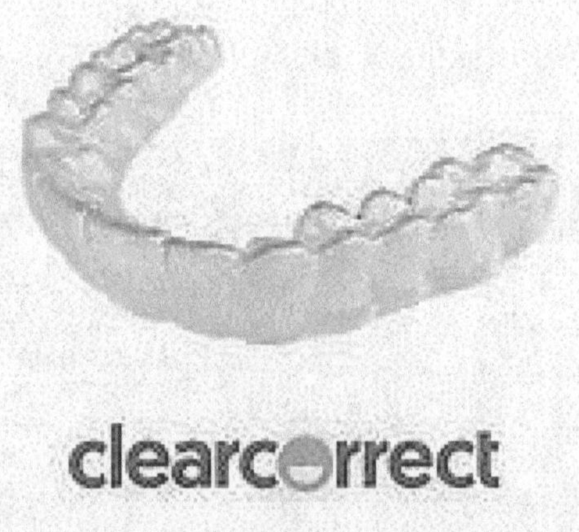

Smile Direct Club

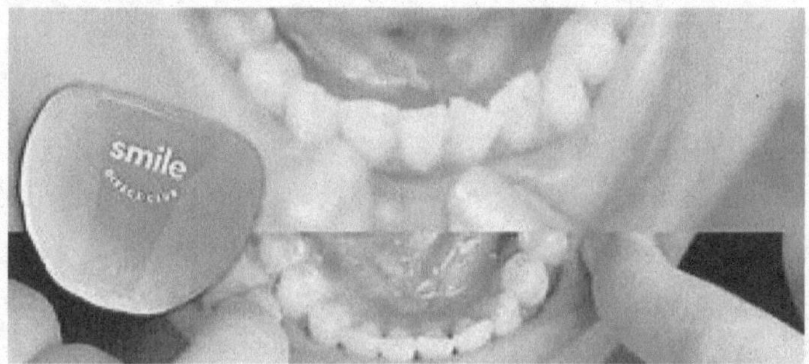

Smile Direct Club (SDC) is a direct-to-consumer (DTC) brand that has grown rapidly by offering a more affordable and convenient option for patients with mild orthodontic issues. Unlike Invisalign and ClearCorrect, SDC does not require regular in-office visits. Patients use an at-home impression kit to get started, and treatment is monitored remotely through virtual check-ins. While the cost is significantly lower, the treatment is primarily designed for minor crowding and spacing issues, limiting its effectiveness for more complex cases.

Other Brands

Several other brands have entered the clear aligner market, each with unique approaches. Brands like Candid, Byte, and ALIGNERCO offer a mix of in-office and DTC options, some focusing on faster treatment timelines using specialized technologies like HyperByte™ (vibration therapy) or AI-driven modeling. These brands vary in cost, technology, and level of supervision, making them a good choice for patients seeking specific features or more affordable options.

In-Office Aligners vs. Direct-to-Consumer Aligners

The main difference between in-office aligners (e.g., Invisalign, ClearCorrect) and DTC aligners (e.g., Smile Direct Club, Byte) lies in the level of professional supervision and the complexity of cases they can treat. In-office aligners involve regular visits to a dental professional, who can make real-time adjustments and address any complications.

This makes them more suitable for complex cases, including bite corrections and severe crowding.

On the other hand, DTC aligners offer convenience and affordability by allowing patients to manage their treatment from home with remote supervision. However, this model is better suited for minor adjustments and requires patients to be disciplined in following instructions without close professional monitoring.

Suitability for Different Types of Dental Corrections

Choosing the right clear aligner depends largely on the type and severity of the dental correction needed.

For complex cases involving significant bite adjustments, crowding, or spacing, in-office treatments like Invisalign or ClearCorrect are more reliable due to the high level of customization and professional oversight. For mild cases, where convenience and affordability are key factors, DTC options like Smile Direct Club or Byte can be effective solutions.

Chapter 4

Advantages of Clear Aligners

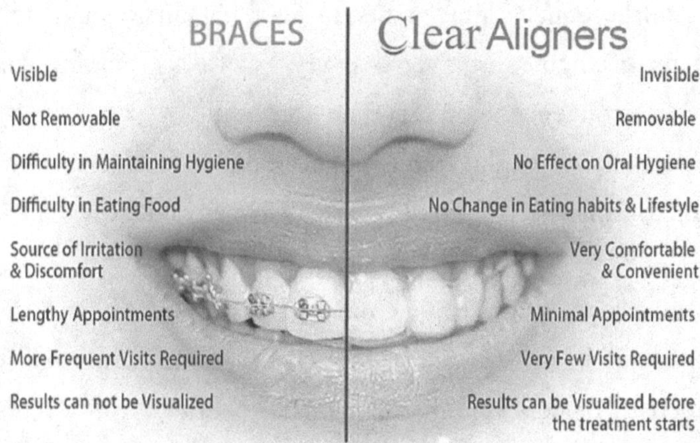

1. Aesthetic Appeal and Invisibility

Clear aligners are crafted from transparent plastic, making them virtually invisible when worn. This feature is especially advantageous for adults and teens who may be self-conscious about the appearance of metal braces. Unlike traditional braces, which are noticeable and can impact a person's smile, clear aligners blend seamlessly with the natural teeth. This aesthetic benefit allows patients to undergo orthodontic treatment with minimal impact on their everyday appearance and social interactions. The discrete nature of clear aligners means patients can confidently smile and speak without feeling self-conscious.

2. Comfort and Convenience

Clear aligners are designed to provide a comfortable fit with minimal disruption to daily life. The aligners are made from smooth, flexible plastic, which reduces the likelihood of irritation or injury to the inside of the mouth and gums. Traditional braces often involve brackets and wires that can cause sores or discomfort. In contrast, clear aligners are custom-made for each patient, ensuring a snug and gentle fit. Additionally, aligners do not require frequent adjustments; instead, patients typically change to the next set of aligners in a series every 1-2 weeks, making the overall process more convenient and less time-consuming.\

Clear aligners are engineered to enhance patient comfort and minimize disruption to daily life, offering several distinct advantages over traditional braces:

1. Smooth, Flexible Plastic Construction

Clear aligners are crafted from smooth, flexible plastic materials designed to fit comfortably against the teeth and gums. This design minimizes the risk of irritation or injury to the soft tissues in the mouth, which is a common issue with traditional metal braces. Traditional braces involve metal brackets and wires that can cause sores, abrasions, or discomfort as they come into contact with the inside of the mouth. The absence of such hardware in clear aligners ensures a more comfortable experience, reducing the likelihood of mouth sores or irritation.

2. Custom-Made for Precision Fit

Each set of clear aligners is custom-made based on detailed digital scans and impressions of the patient's teeth. This customization ensures a precise and snug fit, allowing the aligners to exert the right amount of pressure for effective tooth movement. The tailored fit contributes to a more comfortable treatment experience, as the aligners align seamlessly with the natural contours of the teeth and mouth. This level of personalization contrasts with traditional braces, where the standard brackets and wires may not conform as closely to individual dental anatomy.

3. Minimal Disruption to Daily Life

Clear aligners are designed to integrate smoothly into daily life. They are removable, allowing patients to take them out for eating, drinking, and cleaning, which reduces the impact on daily routines. Unlike traditional braces, which require dietary adjustments and can interfere with eating and oral hygiene, aligners offer greater flexibility. Patients can maintain their regular eating habits and oral care routines without significant modifications, leading to a more convenient and less disruptive orthodontic experience.

4. Reduced Need for Frequent Adjustments

The treatment with clear aligners generally involves fewer office visits compared to traditional braces. Instead of frequent adjustments to brackets and wires, patients simply progress through a series of aligners, changing to the next set every 1-2 weeks. This streamlined process reduces the number of visits required to the orthodontist, saving time for both the patient and the provider. This reduction in visits also contributes to a more convenient treatment experience, as patients can manage their progress with minimal disruption to their schedules.

5. Lower Risk of Treatment Discomfort

Clear aligners are designed to exert gentle, consistent pressure on the teeth to achieve gradual movement. This gentle approach reduces the risk of significant discomfort or pain that can occur with the more abrupt pressure of traditional braces. Patients may experience some initial pressure or tightness when switching to a new set of aligners, but this is generally mild and short-lived compared to the potential discomfort of traditional orthodontic adjustments.

6. Enhanced Aesthetic Appeal

The transparent material of clear aligners makes them nearly invisible, which is a significant advantage for patients concerned about the appearance of their orthodontic treatment. The aesthetic appeal of clear aligners allows patients to undergo treatment without the noticeable appearance of metal braces. This aspect enhances the comfort of patients who may feel self-conscious about their appearance during the treatment process.

7. Convenience in Lifestyle Integration

Clear aligners adapt well to various lifestyle needs. For patients with busy schedules or active lives, the convenience of removable aligners means they can continue participating in their preferred activities without hindrance. Whether it's playing a musical instrument, engaging in sports, or attending social events, aligners can be easily removed and replaced, ensuring that the orthodontic treatment does not interfere with daily activities.

8. Ease of Maintenance

Maintaining clear aligners is straightforward. Patients are instructed to clean their aligners with a soft toothbrush and lukewarm water, avoiding abrasive cleaners and hot water that could distort the plastic. The simplicity of cleaning and maintaining the aligners contributes to their overall convenience, ensuring they remain hygienic and effective throughout the treatment period.

9. Improved Oral Hygiene Practices

With clear aligners, patients can maintain regular oral hygiene practices without the obstruction of braces. They can brush and floss their teeth as usual, leading to better overall dental health. The ability to remove aligners during oral care routines helps prevent plaque buildup and reduces the risk of dental issues that are sometimes associated with traditional braces.

10. Personalized Comfort Adjustments

The ability to tailor the aligners to each patient's unique dental needs means that any necessary adjustments for comfort can be easily addressed. Orthodontists can fine-tune the aligners to ensure optimal fit and function, further enhancing the overall comfort and effectiveness of the treatment.

In summary, clear aligners offer significant comfort and convenience advantages over traditional braces. Their smooth, flexible design, custom fit, minimal need for adjustments, and removable nature contribute to a more comfortable and adaptable orthodontic experience. These benefits make clear aligners an attractive option for patients seeking an effective yet unobtrusive method of achieving their orthodontic goals.

3. Removability and Oral Hygiene Maintenance

One of the standout benefits of clear aligners is their removability. Patients can easily take out the aligners during meals, allowing them to eat their favorite foods without restrictions. This is a significant improvement over traditional braces, which often require dietary adjustments to avoid damaging the braces. Additionally, the ability to remove the aligners facilitates better oral hygiene. Patients can brush and floss their teeth without the obstruction of brackets and wires, which helps prevent plaque buildup and maintains overall dental health. Regular cleaning of the aligners themselves is straightforward, requiring just brushing with a toothbrush and rinsing with water. One of the most compelling benefits of clear aligners is their removability, which offers several key advantages over traditional braces. This feature significantly enhances the patient experience in several important ways:

I. Freedom During Meals

Clear aligners can be easily removed during meals, allowing patients to enjoy a wide variety of foods without restrictions. This is a substantial improvement over traditional metal braces, which often require patients to avoid certain foods that could damage the brackets or become trapped in the wires. Sticky candies, popcorn, nuts, and hard foods are common dietary restrictions associated with braces. With clear aligners, patients can remove their aligners before eating, thus avoiding these restrictions and enjoying their favorite foods without worry. This freedom contributes to a more pleasant and less restrictive eating experience.

II. Improved Oral Hygiene

The removability of clear aligners also facilitates superior oral hygiene compared to traditional braces. With braces, the brackets and wires can obstruct thorough brushing and flossing, making it challenging to maintain good oral health. Food particles and plaque can accumulate around the brackets, increasing the risk of dental issues such as cavities and gum disease. Clear aligners, on the other hand, are taken out during brushing and flossing, allowing patients to clean their teeth thoroughly without obstruction. This ease of access helps in preventing plaque buildup and maintaining overall dental health, contributing to a healthier mouth throughout the treatment process.

III. Simplified Cleaning of Aligners

Cleaning clear aligners is straightforward and requires minimal effort. Patients are advised to brush their aligners with a soft toothbrush and rinse them with lukewarm water regularly. This simple maintenance routine helps to keep the aligners free from stains and odors. Unlike braces, which can trap food particles and require special cleaning products, aligners can be easily maintained with routine brushing and rinsing. Regular cleaning ensures that the aligners remain clear and unobtrusive, maintaining their aesthetic appeal throughout the treatment.

IV. Enhanced Comfort and Convenience

The ability to remove aligners contributes to greater comfort and convenience. Traditional braces can sometimes cause irritation or soreness due to the constant presence of metal brackets and wires in the mouth. Clear aligners, being smooth and removable, reduce such discomfort. Patients can also take out their aligners for important occasions, such as social events or presentations, without feeling self-conscious about their orthodontic appliances. This flexibility enhances overall patient satisfaction and makes the orthodontic experience more adaptable to individual lifestyles.

V. Better Management of Special Situations

Clear aligners provide an advantage in managing special situations or emergencies. For instance, if a patient needs to undergo a dental procedure, such as a teeth cleaning or a filling, they can simply remove their aligners. This ease of removal allows for uninterrupted access to the teeth and facilitates any necessary dental work. Traditional braces might complicate such procedures, as the brackets and wires could be in the way or need to be adjusted temporarily.

VI. Support for Active Lifestyles

For individuals who lead active lifestyles or participate in contact sports, clear aligners offer a safer and more convenient option. Unlike braces, which can pose a risk of injury to the mouth and gums during physical activities, aligners can be removed before engaging in sports or strenuous activities. This reduces the risk of oral injuries and allows for a more comfortable and secure fit during active pursuits.

VII. **Reduced Risk of Food Debris**

Because aligners are removed during meals, there is less risk of food debris getting stuck in the orthodontic appliances. This reduction in trapped food particles lowers the likelihood of bad breath and maintains better overall oral hygiene. With traditional braces, food debris can easily become lodged around the brackets and wires, requiring extra effort to clean thoroughly.

VIII. **Flexibility in Personal Care Routines**

Patients with clear aligners benefit from the flexibility to adapt their personal care routines. They can choose when to remove their aligners for eating, drinking, or cleaning, which allows for better integration into their daily lives. This level of control helps patients adhere to their orthodontic treatment plan more comfortably and consistently.

IX. In summary, the removability of clear aligners provides significant benefits, including freedom during meals, improved oral hygiene, easy aligner cleaning, and enhanced comfort. This feature makes clear aligners a more convenient and adaptable orthodontic solution, supporting better oral health and offering a more flexible treatment experience compared to traditional braces.

4. Predictable Outcomes with Digital Planning

Clear aligners benefit from advanced digital technology that enhances the precision and predictability of treatment. Orthodontists use 3D scanning and computer modeling to create a detailed treatment plan, which shows a virtual simulation of how the teeth will move throughout the treatment. This digital planning allows patients to see a preview of their final results before starting the treatment. The use of this technology ensures that the treatment process is more accurate and tailored to the individual needs of each patient. It also allows for adjustments to be made in real-time if needed, further enhancing the predictability and effectiveness of the treatment.

Clear aligners have revolutionized orthodontic treatment with their reliance on cutting-edge digital technology. This advancement significantly enhances the precision, predictability, and customization of orthodontic care. Here's a detailed look at how these technologies contribute to effective clear aligner treatments:

- **3D Scanning Technology**

At the core of clear aligner treatment is 3D scanning technology. This method involves using advanced imaging equipment to capture highly detailed, three-dimensional images of the patient's teeth and oral structures. Unlike traditional impressions, which can be uncomfortable and imprecise, 3D scanning provides an accurate and comfortable alternative. The resulting digital model offers a precise representation of the patient's current dental alignment, setting the foundation for creating a tailored treatment plan.

- **Digital Modeling and Simulation**

Once the 3D scan is completed, digital modeling software comes into play. Orthodontists use sophisticated computer programs to create a virtual model of the patient's teeth. This model enables the simulation of the entire treatment process. By adjusting the virtual teeth positions, orthodontists can visualize and plan how each aligner will progressively shift the teeth into their desired positions. This virtual simulation provides both the orthodontist and the patient with a clear preview of the expected final results, which enhances understanding and sets realistic expectations.

- **Personalized Treatment Planning**

Digital technology allows for highly personalized treatment planning. Orthodontists can use the data from 3D scans and digital models to design aligners that are custom-fit to each patient's unique dental anatomy. This level of customization ensures that each aligner is precisely engineered to apply the correct amount of pressure to specific teeth, facilitating more effective and efficient tooth movement. The result is a treatment plan that is finely tuned to address the individual needs and goals of the patient.

- **Real-Time Adjustments**

One of the significant advantages of digital technology in clear aligner treatment is the ability to make real-time adjustments. If there are any issues or changes in the patient's dental condition during the course of treatment, orthodontists can quickly modify the treatment plan. This might involve updating the digital model and generating new aligners to address any unforeseen complications or adjustments needed for optimal results. This flexibility ensures that the treatment remains on track and can be adapted to changing circumstances.

- **Enhanced Predictability**

The use of digital tools enhances the predictability of treatment outcomes. By visualizing the entire treatment process and potential end results through simulation, both orthodontists and patients gain a better understanding of what to expect. This foresight allows for more accurate planning and reduces the likelihood of surprises during the treatment. The predictability offered by digital planning contributes to higher patient confidence and satisfaction with the overall treatment process.

- **Improved Communication**

Digital technology facilitates better communication between

orthodontists and patients. Detailed visual representations of the treatment plan and progress updates can be shared through digital platforms, making it easier for patients to understand their treatment journey. Clear aligner systems often include patient-friendly software or apps that allow for real-time tracking and communication, ensuring that patients are well-informed and engaged throughout their treatment.

- **Streamlined Production Process**

The integration of digital technology extends to the production of aligners. Once the treatment plan is finalized, the digital model is used to create precise molds for aligner fabrication. Advanced 3D printing techniques are employed to produce aligners with high accuracy and consistency. This streamlined production process not only accelerates the delivery of aligners but also ensures that each set is manufactured to exact specifications.

- **Data-Driven Insights**

Digital tools provide valuable data-driven insights into treatment progress. Orthodontists can track changes and analyze treatment efficacy using data collected from digital scans and monitoring tools. This information helps in evaluating the success of the treatment and making informed decisions about any necessary adjustments.

- In summary, advanced digital technology has transformed clear aligner treatment by enhancing precision, predictability, and customization. 3D scanning and digital modeling create detailed and accurate treatment plans, allowing for virtual simulations and real-time adjustments. This technology ensures that clear aligner treatments are tailored to each patient's needs, leading to more effective and satisfactory outcomes. The improved communication and streamlined production processes further support the overall effectiveness and efficiency of clear aligner therapy.

5. Enhanced Treatment Flexibility

Clear aligners provide a high level of treatment flexibility. Patients have the option to remove their aligners for special occasions or important events, which is not possible with traditional braces. This flexibility allows patients to maintain their lifestyle and participate in activities without feeling restricted. Additionally, clear aligners are typically designed for easier adjustments and modifications, allowing orthodontists to address changes in the treatment plan more conveniently.

Clear aligners offer remarkable flexibility in orthodontic treatment, distinguishing them from traditional metal braces and contributing to a more adaptable and patient-friendly experience. This flexibility manifests in several key ways:

- **Removability for Special Occasions**

One of the most valued aspects of clear aligners is their removability. Patients can take out their aligners for special occasions, such as weddings, parties, or important professional events. This feature is particularly beneficial for individuals who may be self-conscious about their appearance or who want to avoid potential discomfort during such events. Unlike traditional metal braces, which are permanently affixed to the teeth, clear aligners allow patients to enjoy significant moments without the added worry of how their orthodontic appliances might affect their comfort or confidence.

- **Convenience During Meals**

The ability to remove clear aligners during meals is a significant advantage over traditional braces. Patients do not have to restrict their diet to avoid damaging the brackets and wires. They can continue to enjoy a wide range of foods, including those that are sticky, hard, or crunchy, without concern. This flexibility not only enhances the patient's dining experience but also simplifies oral hygiene practices, as aligners are removed, allowing for easier brushing and flossing.

- **Adaptability to Changes in Treatment**

Clear aligner treatment is designed to be highly adaptable. If adjustments to the treatment plan are necessary—whether due to changes in tooth movement, shifts in patient needs, or unforeseen complications—orthodontists can modify the plan and produce new aligners relatively quickly. The digital nature of clear aligner systems allows for real-time updates and precise modifications. This capability ensures that treatment can be tailored more effectively to the patient's evolving orthodontic needs.

- **Streamlined Adjustments and Monitoring**

The process of changing aligners is straightforward and typically involves fewer in-office visits compared to traditional braces. Patients generally switch to a new set of aligners every few weeks as prescribed by their orthodontist. This regular but infrequent change schedule minimizes the need for frequent adjustment appointments, reducing the overall time spent in the orthodontic office. This streamlined approach also means that orthodontists can more easily track progress and make timely modifications to the treatment plan if necessary.

- **Enhanced Lifestyle Integration**

The flexibility of clear aligners supports better integration into the patient's lifestyle. Patients can engage in various activities such as sports, public speaking, or performing arts without the discomfort or potential hazards associated with traditional braces. For example, athletes can remove their aligners during games or practices, reducing the risk of injury that could occur with metal braces. This ease of integration enhances overall patient satisfaction and adherence to the treatment plan.

- **Ease of Oral Hygiene Maintenance**

Maintaining oral hygiene with clear aligners is generally easier than with traditional braces. Since aligners are removable, patients can brush and floss their teeth without obstruction. This ease of access helps prevent plaque buildup, tooth decay, and gum disease, contributing to better overall dental health during orthodontic treatment. The ability to clean teeth thoroughly, along with the convenience of removing aligners for hygiene, further supports patient compliance.

- **Digital Planning and Simulation**

The digital tools used in clear aligner treatment planning offer a high degree of precision and flexibility. Orthodontists can use 3D imaging and modeling to simulate different treatment scenarios and outcomes. This advanced planning allows for more accurate predictions and adjustments, ensuring that treatment can be optimized for the best results. Patients can often see a virtual preview of their expected results before starting treatment, which enhances their understanding and acceptance of the proposed plan.

- **Remote Monitoring Options**

Many clear aligner systems incorporate remote monitoring technology, allowing orthodontists to track treatment progress through digital platforms. Patients can submit photos or updates via apps or online portals, enabling orthodontists to provide feedback and make adjustments without requiring frequent in-person visits. This remote capability offers added convenience and supports more flexible management of the treatment process.

6. Fewer Dietary Restrictions

With traditional metal braces, patients face specific dietary restrictions to avoid complications. Foods that are sticky, chewy, or hard can pose significant challenges. Sticky candies, such as caramel or taffy, can adhere to the brackets and wires, making them difficult to clean and potentially causing damage. Popcorn and nuts are problematic due to their hard and crunchy nature, which can break the brackets or bend the wires. Such damage not only prolongs treatment but can also lead to additional discomfort and the need for emergency orthodontic visits to repair or replace broken components.

In contrast, clear aligners offer a significant advantage in this regard. One of the primary benefits of clear aligners is their removability. Patients are instructed to remove their aligners before eating and drinking, which effectively eliminates the risk of food-related damage to the aligners. This flexibility allows patients to enjoy a broader range of foods without the usual concerns associated with traditional braces.

This freedom to eat without restrictions contributes to a more enjoyable and less restrictive eating experience. Patients can savor foods like popcorn, nuts, and sticky candies without having to worry about potential damage to their orthodontic appliances or the need for special cleaning methods. Additionally, since aligners are removed for meals, patients can maintain better oral hygiene. They can brush and floss their teeth without the obstructions of brackets and wires, reducing the risk of plaque buildup and oral health issues.

Furthermore, the absence of dietary restrictions and the ease of maintaining oral hygiene with clear aligners can lead to higher patient satisfaction. This aspect of clear aligner treatment not only enhances comfort but also supports better compliance with treatment protocols. Overall, the ability to enjoy a wider variety of foods and maintain optimal oral hygiene contributes to a more convenient and pleasant orthodontic experience, reinforcing the appeal of clear aligners as a modern alternative to traditional braces.

7. Reduced Treatment Time

For many patients, clear aligners can lead to faster treatment times compared to traditional braces. The precise, digital treatment planning and custom aligner sets allow for efficient tooth movement. While treatment duration varies based on individual needs, some cases with clear aligners can be completed more quickly than with traditional methods. The ability to visualize and adjust the treatment plan with digital tools also contributes to more streamlined and effective treatment.

Faster Treatment Times with Clear Aligners

Clear aligners often offer the advantage of potentially faster treatment times compared to traditional metal braces, thanks to several key factors related to digital technology and treatment efficiency.

A. Precision in Treatment Planning

Clear aligners leverage advanced digital technology for treatment planning. This begins with 3D scanning and digital modeling of the patient's dental anatomy. The precision of these digital tools allows for the creation of a highly accurate treatment plan that maps out the entire course of the orthodontic intervention. By using computer-generated simulations, orthodontists can design a series of aligners that are tailored to achieve optimal tooth movement in the most efficient manner possible. This level of precision minimizes guesswork and ensures that each aligner is designed to move the teeth incrementally toward the desired final position.

B. Custom Aligner Sets

Clear aligners are custom-made for each patient based on the detailed digital treatment plan. Each set of aligners is designed to apply controlled and specific forces to the teeth, facilitating their gradual movement. The customization of each aligner set ensures that the forces applied are optimized for the patient's unique orthodontic needs, potentially leading to more efficient movement and quicker results. This tailored approach contrasts with traditional braces, where adjustments are made manually and might not always account for the precise forces needed at every stage of treatment.

C. Reduced Need for Frequent Adjustments

Traditional metal braces require periodic adjustments by the orthodontist to tighten wires and reposition brackets. These adjustments can be time-consuming and may lead to variable treatment speeds depending on the complexity of the case and the frequency of visits. Clear aligners, however, reduce the need for such frequent in-office adjustments. Once the aligner sets are provided, patients typically switch to a new set of aligners every 1-2 weeks, according to the treatment plan. This streamlined process can reduce the number of orthodontic visits required, contributing to a more efficient overall treatment timeline.

D. Real-Time Treatment Monitoring and Adjustments

Digital treatment planning and monitoring allow for real-time evaluation of progress. Orthodontists can use digital tools to assess how well the treatment is progressing compared to the initial plan. If necessary, adjustments can be made to the treatment plan based on this assessment. This flexibility and ability to make data-driven decisions enhance the efficiency of the treatment process. In contrast, traditional braces often rely on physical observations and manual adjustments, which may not always capture every nuance of progress.

E. Case-Specific Advantages

While treatment duration with clear aligners varies based on individual orthodontic needs, many cases can be completed more quickly than with traditional braces. For patients with mild to moderate orthodontic issues, clear aligners can provide an effective solution in a shorter time frame. The ability to visualize the entire treatment process through digital simulations allows for precise tracking of progress and timely adjustments, potentially accelerating the overall treatment duration.

F. Enhanced Patient Compliance

Clear aligners are removable, which means patients can take them out for eating, drinking, and oral hygiene. This convenience often leads to higher patient compliance compared to traditional braces, where the constraints of brackets and wires can make oral care more challenging. Higher compliance can result in more predictable and efficient treatment outcomes, as patients are more likely to adhere to the prescribed aligner wear schedule and maintain good oral hygiene.

8. Improved Patient Compliance

Clear aligners often lead to better patient compliance due to their convenience and aesthetic benefits. Since the aligners are removable, patients can adhere to the treatment plan more easily without the discomfort or inconvenience of traditional braces. The ability to remove aligners for special occasions or when necessary can also improve patient satisfaction and willingness to follow through with the treatment. This increased compliance often results in more successful outcomes and a smoother treatment process.

Clear aligners have gained popularity not only for their effectiveness in treating orthodontic issues but also for the advantages they offer in terms of patient compliance. Several key factors contribute to this enhanced compliance, driven primarily by the convenience and aesthetic benefits of clear aligners.

- **Removability and Convenience**

One of the most significant benefits of clear aligners is their removability. Unlike traditional metal braces, which are fixed to the teeth and require patients to adjust their eating and oral hygiene habits, clear aligners can be taken out as needed. This feature allows patients to eat and drink without restrictions, which can significantly impact their overall satisfaction with the treatment. The ability to remove aligners makes it easier to maintain normal eating habits, avoid food-related issues, and enjoy a wider variety of foods without the worry of damaging the orthodontic appliances.

- **Aesthetic Appeal**

Clear aligners are designed to be nearly invisible when worn, making them a more discreet option compared to traditional metal braces. This aesthetic advantage is particularly appealing to adults and teenagers who may be self-conscious about their appearance during orthodontic treatment. The invisibility of clear aligners helps patients feel more confident and less concerned about the impact of their braces on their social interactions and professional image. This increased self-esteem can positively influence their willingness to adhere to the treatment plan.

- **Flexibility for Special Occasions**

The removability of clear aligners also offers flexibility for special occasions or situations where patients might prefer not to wear their aligners. For instance, patients can remove their aligners for important events such as weddings, interviews, or social gatherings, which can significantly enhance their comfort and confidence. This flexibility reduces the potential for discomfort or self-consciousness that might otherwise affect their commitment to the treatment plan.

- **Improved Oral Hygiene**

Maintaining oral hygiene is often more straightforward with clear aligners compared to traditional braces. Since aligners are removable, patients can brush and floss their teeth more easily, without the need to navigate around brackets and wires. Good oral hygiene is crucial during orthodontic treatment to prevent plaque buildup, tooth decay, and gum issues. The ability to maintain effective oral care can lead to better overall dental health and fewer complications, contributing to a more positive treatment experience.

- **Clear Aligner Adjustments and Monitoring**

Clear aligner systems typically involve fewer in-office adjustments compared to traditional braces. Patients follow a treatment plan that involves changing to a new set of aligners every few weeks. The process is relatively straightforward, and many patients find it easier to manage compared to the frequent adjustments and tightening appointments required with metal braces. This simplified approach can lead to higher compliance as patients are less likely to miss appointments or feel overwhelmed by frequent adjustments.

- **Digital Monitoring and Feedback**

Many clear aligner systems incorporate digital tools that allow for remote monitoring and virtual consultations. Patients can often use apps or online platforms to upload progress photos, receive feedback from their orthodontists, and track their treatment. This digital engagement provides ongoing support and guidance, helping patients stay on track and address any concerns promptly. The convenience of digital monitoring can further enhance compliance and contribute to a smoother treatment process.

- **Positive Reinforcement and Motivation**

The aesthetic benefits and flexibility of clear aligners often lead to increased patient satisfaction, which can serve as positive reinforcement for adherence to the treatment plan. When patients see the progress they are making and experience fewer disruptions to their daily lives, they are more likely to remain motivated and committed to completing the treatment. This intrinsic motivation can lead to higher compliance rates and better overall outcomes.

Advantage	Description
Aesthetic Appeal and Invisibility	Clear aligners are made from transparent plastic, making them nearly invisible when worn. This is especially appealing to those who prefer a discreet orthodontic solution.
Comfort and Convenience	Clear aligners are smooth and flexible, reducing irritation compared to metal braces. They are custom-fitted and easy to insert and remove, minimizing disruption to daily life.
Removability and Oral Hygiene Maintenance	Aligners can be removed for eating and cleaning, allowing for easier oral hygiene and a wider variety of foods. This prevents plaque buildup and maintains better dental health.
Predictable Outcomes with Digital Planning	Advanced 3D scanning and digital modeling provide precise treatment planning and visual simulations of expected results. This ensures accuracy and helps patients see the final outcome before starting.
Enhanced Treatment Flexibility	Patients can remove aligners for special occasions or important events, offering flexibility that is not available with traditional braces.

Fewer Dietary Restrictions	Unlike traditional braces, aligners can be removed during meals, allowing patients to eat a variety of foods without restrictions or damage to the orthodontic appliances.
Reduced Treatment Time	The precise and efficient digital treatment planning can lead to faster overall treatment times for many patients compared to traditional braces.
Improved Patient Compliance	The convenience and aesthetics of clear aligners often lead to better adherence to the treatment plan, resulting in more successful outcomes.

Chapter 5

Limitations and Challenges

Clear aligners have revolutionized orthodontic treatment, but they come with their own set of limitations and challenges. Let's explore these in detail with illustrative examples to provide a clearer understanding.

1. Not Suitable for All Cases: Complex Malocclusions and Severe Crowding

Example: Esha's Severe Overbite

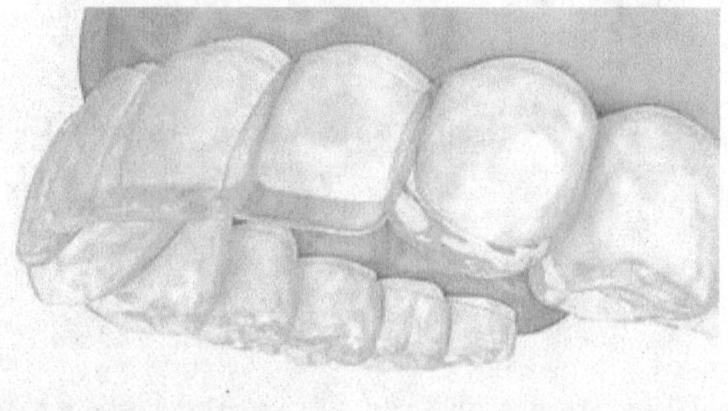

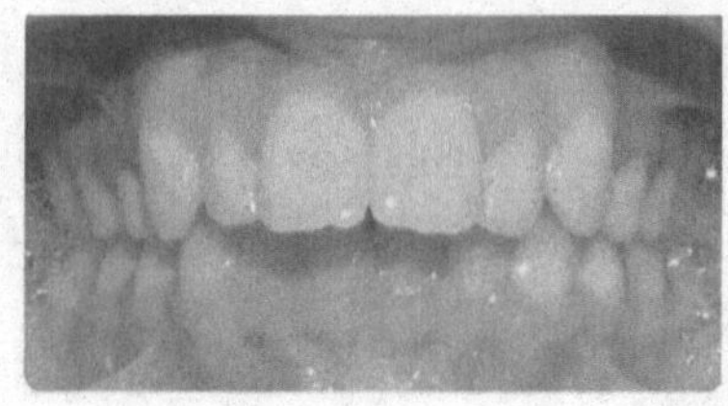
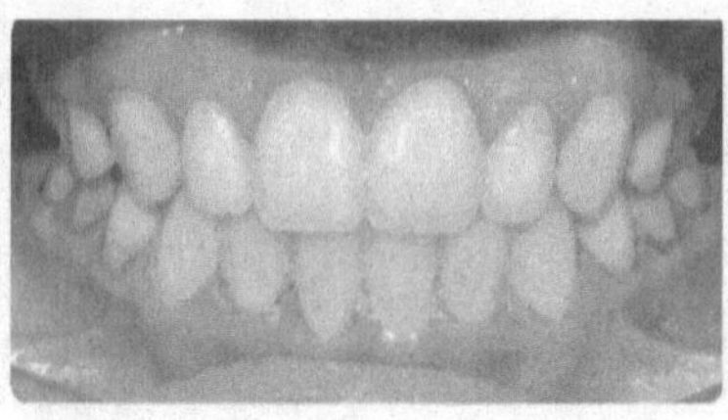

Esha, a 28-year-old professional, sought orthodontic treatment for her severe overbite and significant crowding. Her teeth were so crowded that some were overlapping and not in line, while her overbite was causing functional issues. Clear aligners were initially recommended, but upon further examination, it was determined that her case was too complex for aligners alone. The orthodontist advised that traditional metal braces, or possibly even surgical intervention, would be more effective in addressing the severe crowding and overbite, as they can provide more precise control and apply stronger forces to move the teeth into proper alignment.

Example: Jagjeet Complex Crossbite

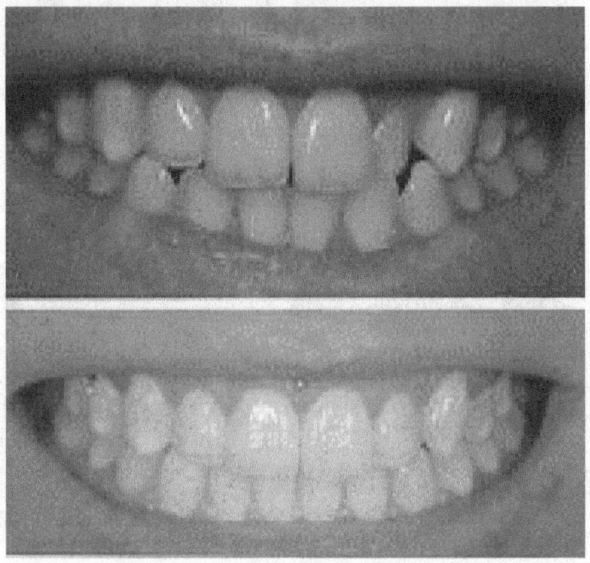

Jagjeet, a 35-year-old with a complex crossbite, where his upper teeth were significantly misaligned with his lower teeth, also faced challenges with clear aligners. His orthodontist explained that the severity of his crossbite required the use of metal braces or other orthodontic appliances to achieve the necessary tooth movement and correct the bite effectively. Clear aligners would not have been able to provide the precise adjustments needed for his condition.

2. Cost Considerations

Example: Sakshi's Budget Constraints

Sakshi, a college student, was excited about the prospect of clear aligners due to their aesthetic appeal. However, when she learned about the cost, which was significantly higher than traditional braces, she faced a dilemma. The advanced technology involved in clear aligner treatment led to higher expenses, and her dental insurance plan only covered a portion of the cost. To manage her budget, Sakshi considered traditional braces, which were more affordable and covered more comprehensively by her insurance. She had to weigh the benefits of clear aligners against her financial constraints.

Example: Manish's Financial Planning

Manish, a 45-year-old professional with a high-paying job, was interested in clear aligners for their convenience and aesthetic benefits. Despite having the financial means to afford the higher cost, he still needed to evaluate whether the investment aligned with his long-term goals. He explored various payment options, including flexible financing plans offered by his orthodontist, to make the cost of clear aligners more manageable.

3. Compliance and Patient Discipline

Example: Latikha Struggle with Consistency

Latikha, a 22-year-old student, was enthusiastic about using clear aligners but struggled with compliance. She often forgot to wear her aligners for the recommended 20-22 hours per day, and frequently took them out for social events and meals. Her orthodontist warned that inconsistent wear could extend her treatment time and reduce the effectiveness of the aligners. Latikha's experience highlighted the importance of discipline and adherence to the treatment plan for achieving the desired results with clear aligners.

Example: Tomar's Challenges with Aligner Changes

Tomar, a 30-year-old professional, found it challenging to keep track of when to switch to the next set of aligners. He sometimes missed the scheduled change dates, which led to delays in his treatment progress. His orthodontist emphasized the need for strict adherence to the aligner schedule to ensure proper tooth movement and avoid complications. Tomar's situation underscored the necessity of patient discipline and proper management of the treatment plan.

4. Potential for Discomfort and Temporary Side Effects

Example: Ekta Initial Discomfort

Ekta, a 25-year-old graphic designer, experienced some discomfort during the initial days of wearing her clear aligners. She felt pressure on her teeth and had a mild lisp when speaking. Although these side effects were temporary and subsided as she adjusted to the aligners, Ekta found them uncomfortable at first. Her orthodontist assured her that such discomfort was normal and would diminish as the aligners began to fit more comfortably.

Example: Dwivedi's Gum Irritation

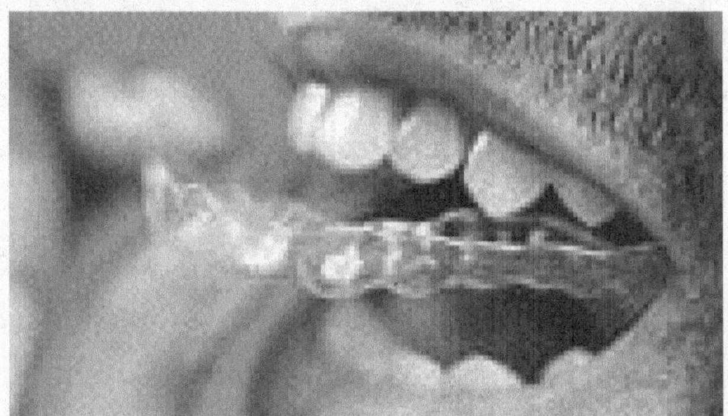

Dwivedi, a 40-year-old lawyer, noticed mild irritation on his gums and the inside of his cheeks after starting clear aligner treatment. The aligners initially caused some soreness and minor sores, which were temporary and resolved as he became accustomed to the aligners. His orthodontist advised using orthodontic wax and maintaining good oral hygiene to minimize irritation and discomfort during the adjustment period.

Summary

While clear aligners offer a range of benefits, including aesthetics and comfort, they are not without limitations. They may not be suitable for all orthodontic cases, can be costly, require strict patient compliance, and may cause temporary discomfort. Understanding these challenges, through real-life examples, helps patients and practitioners make informed decisions and set realistic expectations for orthodontic treatment.

Chapter 6

Patient Experience and Journey

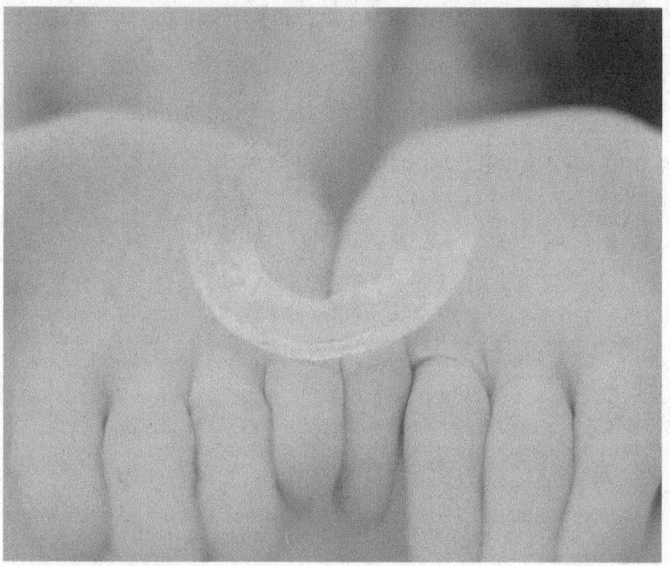

Orthodontic treatment with clear aligners involves more than just wearing a series of plastic trays. It encompasses a comprehensive patient journey, from the initial consultation through the final stages of treatment and beyond. This chapter explores the entire patient experience, including the initial consultation, treatment timeline, management of common issues, and the crucial retention phase.

Initial Consultation and Diagnosis

The First Meeting

The initial consultation is a critical step in the clear aligner journey. During this meeting, the orthodontist or dental professional evaluates the patient's dental and orthodontic needs to determine if clear aligners are a suitable treatment option. This process typically involves several key components:

1. **Patient History and Goals**: The orthodontist begins by discussing the patient's dental history, current issues, and treatment goals. This helps in understanding the patient's concerns and expectations.

2. **Clinical Examination**: A thorough clinical examination is conducted, which includes assessing the alignment of the teeth, the bite, and any potential complications. This examination helps identify the specific orthodontic issues that need to be addressed.

3. **Diagnostic Records**: To create an accurate treatment plan, diagnostic records are gathered. These may include digital X-rays, photographs of the teeth and face, and impressions or scans of the teeth. Modern practices often use 3D scanning technology to create a precise digital model of the patient's dental structure.

4. **Treatment Plan Discussion**: Once the diagnostic records are analyzed, the orthodontist discusses potential treatment options with the patient. If clear aligners are deemed appropriate, the orthodontist explains how the aligners will address the specific orthodontic issues.

Example: Sakshi's Consultation

Sakshi's, a 27-year-old graphic designer, visited her orthodontist with concerns about mild spacing and crooked teeth. After a thorough examination and digital scanning, her orthodontist determined that clear aligners were a suitable option for her case. The orthodontist explained how the aligners would gradually shift her teeth into the desired position, and Sarah was excited to start the treatment.

Understanding the Treatment Timeline

Phases of Treatment

The clear aligner treatment timeline can vary depending on the complexity of the case, but it generally follows a structured process:

1. **Preparation**: After the initial consultation, a detailed treatment plan is created using 3D modeling technology. This plan includes a series of aligners customized for the patient's specific needs. The treatment plan also provides a projected timeline for the entire process.

2. **Receiving the Aligners**: Once the aligners are manufactured, the patient receives a series of aligners, each designed to be worn for a specific duration, typically 1-2 weeks. The orthodontist provides instructions on how to wear and care for the aligners.

3. **Monitoring Progress**: Regular check-ups are scheduled throughout the treatment to monitor progress and make any necessary adjustments. These visits allow the orthodontist to ensure that the aligners are working as intended and to address any concerns the patient may have.

4. **Completion and Final Assessment**: Upon completing the aligner series, the orthodontist evaluates the final results. If the treatment goals have been met, the patient is transitioned to the retention phase. If additional adjustments are needed, the orthodontist may provide additional aligners.

Example: Tomar's Treatment Timeline

Tomar, a 33-year-old marketing manager, started his clear aligner treatment with an estimated timeline of 12 months. His treatment plan included 24 sets of aligners, with each set to be worn for two weeks. Regular check-ups every six to eight weeks allowed his orthodontist to monitor his progress and make adjustments as needed.

Dealing with Discomfort, Lisping, and Oral Hygiene Tips

Managing Discomfort

While clear aligners are generally more comfortable than traditional braces, patients may experience some discomfort as their teeth shift into place. Here's how to manage it:

1. **Initial Pressure**: Patients may feel pressure or slight pain when first wearing a new set of aligners. This is a normal part of the adjustment process. Over-the-counter pain relievers, such as ibuprofen, can help alleviate discomfort.

2. **Gum Irritation**: Some patients may experience irritation or soreness in the gums or the inside of the cheeks. Using orthodontic wax on the edges of the aligners can help soothe these areas.

Example: Esha's Discomfort

Esha, a 25-year-old student, experienced mild discomfort during the first few days of wearing her new aligners. She used pain relievers as recommended by her orthodontist and applied orthodontic wax to reduce gum irritation. By the end of the week, the discomfort had subsided, and she felt more comfortable with her aligners.

Managing Lisping

A temporary lisp is a common side effect when patients first start using clear aligners. This occurs because the aligners can affect speech patterns. Most patients adjust to this within a few days to weeks. Practicing speaking exercises and reading aloud can help expedite this adjustment period.

Example: Dwivedi's Lisp

Dwivedi, a 40-year-old lawyer, noticed a slight lisp when he began using his aligners. He practiced speaking exercises and read aloud to help improve his speech clarity. Within a week, his lisp diminished, and he felt more confident speaking with his aligners.

Oral Hygiene Tips

Maintaining good oral hygiene is essential during clear aligner treatment. Here are some tips:

1. **Regular Brushing and Flossing**: Brush and floss your teeth after every meal to remove food particles and prevent plaque buildup. This is crucial since aligners can trap food and bacteria against the teeth.

2. **Cleaning Aligners**: Rinse aligners with lukewarm water and brush them gently with a soft toothbrush. Avoid using hot water or harsh cleaning agents that can damage the aligners.

3. **Avoid Sugary Drinks**: Remove aligners before drinking sugary beverages, as they can contribute to tooth decay. Water is the best choice while wearing aligners.

Example: Latikha's Hygiene Routine

Latikha, a 22-year-old college student, was diligent about her oral hygiene during her clear aligner treatment. She brushed and flossed her teeth after every meal and cleaned her aligners daily with a soft toothbrush and mild soap. Her commitment to maintaining good oral hygiene helped her avoid issues such as tooth decay and plaque buildup.

Retention Phase: The Importance of Retainers Post-Treatment

Why Retainers are Necessary

After completing clear aligner treatment, the retention phase is crucial for maintaining the results achieved. Retainers help ensure that the teeth remain in their new positions and do not shift back to their original alignment. Here's why retainers are important:

1. **Teeth Stability**: Even after the aligners have shifted the teeth into the desired positions, the surrounding bone and tissue need time to stabilize and adapt. Retainers help keep the teeth in place during this stabilization period.

2. **Preventing Relapse**: Without retainers, there is a risk of the teeth

gradually moving back to their original positions. Wearing retainers as prescribed helps prevent this relapse and ensures the longevity of the treatment results.

Types of Retainers

1. **Fixed Retainers**: These are thin wires bonded to the back of the teeth, typically used for the lower front teeth. They provide constant, discreet support and are effective in preventing relapse.

2. **Removable Retainers**: These are custom-made clear or plastic devices that patients can take in and out. They are worn according to the orthodontist's instructions, which may vary from full-time to part-time wear.

Example: Sakshi"s Retainer Use

Sakshi'h, who completed her clear aligner treatment, was provided with a removable retainer to wear at night. Her orthodontist instructed her to use it consistently for the first few months and then gradually reduce usage based on her progress. Sarah adhered to the retainer schedule, which helped her maintain the results of her treatment.

Summary

The patient experience with clear aligners involves several stages, from the initial consultation and diagnosis to managing the treatment process and transitioning into the retention phase. Understanding the treatment timeline, dealing with common issues such as discomfort and lisping, and maintaining good oral hygiene are crucial for a successful orthodontic journey. The retention phase plays a vital role in preserving the results achieved and ensuring long-term satisfaction with clear aligner treatment. By following these guidelines and working closely with their orthodontist, patients can achieve a beautifully aligned smile and enjoy the benefits of clear aligners.

Table summarizing the key points of Chapter 6: Patient Experience and Journey

Aspect	Details
Initial Consultation and Diagnosis	- **Patient History and Goals**: Discuss dental history and treatment goals. - **Clinical Examination**: Assess teeth alignment, bite, and potential issues. - **Diagnostic Records**: Collect digital X-rays, photographs, and impressions. - **Treatment Plan Discussion**: Explain clear aligner treatment if suitable.
Example: Sakshi's Consultation	Sakshi had mild spacing and crooked teeth. After a digital scan, clear aligners were chosen as her treatment.
Understanding the Treatment Timeline	- **Preparation**: Create a detailed treatment plan with 3D modeling. - **Receiving Aligners**: Get a series of aligners to be worn for 1-2 weeks each. - **Monitoring Progress**: Regular check-ups to adjust treatment. - **Completion and Final Assessment**: Evaluate results and transition to retention.
Example: Tomar's Treatment Timeline	Tomar's treatment involved 24 aligners over 12 months, with regular check-ups every 6-8 weeks.
Dealing with Discomfort, Lisping, and Oral Hygiene Tips	- **Managing Discomfort**: Use pain relievers and orthodontic wax. - **Managing Lisping**: Practice speaking exercises. - **Oral Hygiene Tips**: Brush and floss after meals; clean aligners daily; avoid sugary drinks.
Example: Esha's Discomfort	Esha experienced initial discomfort and used pain relievers and wax. The discomfort

	subsided within a week.
Example: Dwivedi's Lisp	Dwivedi had a temporary lisp that improved with speaking exercises.
Retention Phase: The Importance of Retainers Post-Treatment	- **Need for Retainers**: Maintain teeth positions and prevent relapse. - **Types of Retainers**: Fixed (bonded wire) and Removable (clear or plastic).
Example: Sakshi's Retainer Use	Sakshi was provided with a removable retainer to wear at night and followed the orthodontist's instructions.

Chapter 7

Clinical Applications and Case Studies

- Clear aligners have demonstrated their effectiveness in addressing a variety of orthodontic issues. This chapter delves into clinical applications through case studies, showcasing how clear aligners handle different types of dental corrections. We also explore before-and-after results, the role of orthodontists and specialists, and share patient testimonials and success stories.

Case Studies: Mild Crowding, Spacing, Overbite, and Underbite Corrections

1. Mild Crowding

Case Study: Eshwari Transformation

- **Patient Profile**: Eshwari, a 24-year-old graphic designer, presented with mild crowding in the lower front teeth.

- **Treatment Plan**: Eshwari 's orthodontist recommended clear aligners to address the slight overlap and create space for better alignment.

- **Results**: Over a 10-month period, Eshwari wore a series of 20 aligners, with progress monitored at regular intervals. Her teeth were straightened effectively, and the crowding was resolved, resulting in a more aesthetically pleasing smile.

2. Spacing

Case Study: Amit's Spacing Issue

- **Patient Profile**: Amit, a 30-year-old accountant, had noticeable gaps between his upper front teeth.

- **Treatment Plan**: Clear aligners were chosen to gradually close the gaps and align the teeth. The treatment involved a series of 18 aligners over 8 months.
- **Results**: The gaps were successfully closed, and the alignment improved significantly, enhancing both function and appearance.

3. Overbite

Case Study: Lakshami's Overbite Correction

- **Patient Profile**: Lakshami, a 26-year-old nurse, had a moderate overbite where her upper teeth significantly overlapped her lower teeth.
- **Treatment Plan**: The orthodontist used clear aligners along with some interproximal reduction to address the overbite. The treatment lasted for 12 months with 24 aligners.
- **Results**: Lakshami's overbite was corrected, resulting in a more balanced bite and improved smile aesthetics. Her teeth alignment also contributed to better oral function.

4. Underbite

Case Study: Mohinder's Underbite Resolution

- **Patient Profile**: Mohinder, a 32-year-old teacher, presented with a mild underbite where his lower teeth were positioned ahead of the upper teeth.
- **Treatment Plan**: Clear aligners were used to gradually reposition the lower teeth and improve the bite. The treatment was extended to 14 months with 28 aligners.
- **Results**: The underbite was significantly improved, and Mohinder experienced enhanced chewing function and a more harmonious smile.

Before-and-After Results of Clear Aligner Treatments

Example: Eshwari's Case

- **Before**: Mild crowding in the lower front teeth, with noticeable overlap.

- **After**: Teeth were aligned with no crowding. The overall smile appeared straighter and more even.

Example: Amit's Case

- **Before**: Gaps between upper front teeth.

- **After**: Gaps were closed, resulting in a more cohesive and aesthetically pleasing alignment.

Example: Lakshami's Case

- **Before**: Moderate overbite with significant upper teeth overlap.

- **After**: Overbite corrected, teeth alignment improved, and smile aesthetics enhanced.

Example: Mohinder's Case

- **Before**: Mild underbite with lower teeth ahead of upper teeth.

- **After**: Underbite improved, with better alignment and a more balanced bite.

Role of Orthodontists and Specialists in Clear Aligner Therapy

Orthodontists

Orthodontists play a crucial role in the clear aligner therapy process:

1. **Diagnosis and Treatment Planning**: Orthodontists assess the patient's dental needs, create a customized treatment plan, and use digital tools to map out the aligner treatment.

2. **Monitoring Progress**: Regular check-ups are essential to ensure the aligners are working as planned and to make necessary adjustments.

3. **Addressing Complex Cases**: For more challenging cases, orthodontists might combine clear aligners with other orthodontic

tools or therapies.

Specialists

In some cases, other dental specialists may be involved:

1. **Oral Surgeons**: For complex cases requiring surgical intervention, oral surgeons collaborate with orthodontists to ensure comprehensive treatment.

2. **Periodontists**: If a patient has gum issues, periodontists may work alongside orthodontists to address these concerns before or during aligner treatment.

Patient Testimonials and Success Stories

1. Eshwari's Experience

Jenna, 24, shares: "I was hesitant about clear aligners at first, but the results have been fantastic. The process was smooth, and my confidence has grown with my new smile."

2. Amit's Feedback

Alex, 30, says: "The aligners worked perfectly for my spacing issues. I loved that they were virtually invisible, and I could see the improvements as I progressed through each set."

3. Lakshami's Review

Laura, 26, comments: "The treatment was longer than I anticipated, but the outcome was worth it. My bite feels much better, and my smile looks great!"

4. Mohinder's Testimonial

Mark, 32, states: "I had a mild underbite for years, and clear aligners made a huge difference. The treatment was comfortable, and the results exceeded my expectations."

Summary

Clear aligners have proven effective in treating a variety of orthodontic issues, including mild crowding, spacing, overbite, and underbite. Case studies demonstrate their ability to improve dental alignment and overall smile aesthetics. Orthodontists and specialists play essential roles in the treatment process, ensuring that patients receive personalized and effective care. Patient testimonials highlight the success and satisfaction experienced by many individuals who have undergone clear aligner treatment, reflecting its positive impact on both dental health and self-confidence.

Table detailing the clinical applications of clear aligners for various orthodontic problems:

Orthodontic Problem	Case Study Example	Treatment Plan	Treatment Duration	Before-and-After Results	Key Considerations
Mild Crowding	Eshwari, 24, graphic designer	Clear aligners to alleviate slight overlap and create space	10 months, 20 aligners	Teeth straightened with no crowding	Effective for minor crowding; regular monitoring needed
Spacing	Amit, 30, accountant	Clear aligners to close gaps between upper front teeth	8 months, 18 aligners	Gaps closed, improved alignment	Suitable for moderate spacing; requires precise aligner fit
Moderate Overbite	Lakshami, 26, nurse	Clear aligners combined with interproximal	12 months, 24 aligners	Overbite corrected, improved smile aesthetics	Effective for moderate cases; may need additional adjustments

		reduction to correct overbite			
Mild Underbite	Mohinder, 32, teacher	Clear aligners to reposition lower teeth and improve bite	14 months, 28 aligners	Underbite improved, balanced bite achieved	Suitable for mild underbites; may require longer treatment
Severe Crowding	Ekta, 29, lawyer	Clear aligners combined with extractions or interproximal reduction	18 months, 36 aligners	Significant crowding reduced, better alignment	May need additional orthodontic tools or procedures
Severe Spacing	Jasbeer, 40, IT specialist	Clear aligners with attachments to close large gaps	12 months, 24 aligners	Large gaps closed, teeth aligned	Requires careful planning; attachments aid in gap closure
Deep Overbite	Raichandani, 35, teacher	Clear aligners with vertical dimension correction	16 months, 32 aligners	Deep overbite reduced, improved bite function	Complex cases; may need complementary treatments
Open Bite	Mishrish, 28, engineer	Clear aligners with potential bite blocks	15 months, 30 aligners	Open bite corrected, better occlusion	Requires close monitoring; elastic bands may be

		or elastic bands			necessary
Crossbite	Sakshi, 31, marketing manager	Clear aligners with additional appliances for correction	14 months, 28 aligners	Crossbite corrected, improved alignment	May need auxiliary devices; precise adjustment required
Protruded Teeth	Dwivedi, 27, student	Clear aligners to retract protruded front teeth	12 months, 24 aligners	Protrusion reduced, teeth repositioned	Suitable for moderate protrusion; may need adjustments
Tooth Rotation	Lathika, 23, photographer	Clear aligners with rotation attachments	10 months, 20 aligners	Rotated teeth aligned, improved smile	Attachments used for effective rotation correction
Asymmetric Bite	Keshav, 37, sales executive	Clear aligners to address asymmetric alignment	16 months, 32 aligners	Bite symmetry improved, teeth aligned	Requires detailed planning; results vary based on complexity

Chapter 8

Technological Innovations in Clear Aligners

Technological advancements have significantly enhanced the efficacy and accessibility of clear aligner treatments. This chapter explores key innovations in the field, including advances in 3D printing and material science, the integration of AI and machine learning in treatment planning, the future of teledentistry and at-home aligner systems, and the growing trend of customization and personalization in orthodontic care.

1. Advances in 3D Printing and Aligner Material Science

3D Printing Technology

- **High Precision and Speed**: Advances in 3D printing have revolutionized the production of clear aligners. Modern 3D printers use high-resolution technology to create highly accurate models of patients' teeth. This precision ensures that aligners fit perfectly and work effectively to move teeth into the desired position.

- **Material Innovation**: The development of new 3D printing materials has led to improved aligner durability and comfort. For example, biocompatible resins used in printing are more flexible and resistant to staining, providing better performance and aesthetics.

- **Rapid Prototyping**: 3D printing allows for rapid prototyping and customization of aligners. Orthodontists can quickly create and adjust aligner models based on patient feedback and treatment progress, leading to more efficient and personalized treatment plans.

Example: A patient undergoing treatment with a new resin material may experience enhanced comfort and fewer adjustments due to the improved fit and flexibility of the aligners.

Aligner Material Science

- **Advanced Thermoplastics**: Modern aligners are made from advanced thermoplastics, such as polyurethane and PETG (polyethylene terephthalate glycol). These materials are known for their strength, flexibility, and clarity, providing a comfortable and nearly invisible option for patients.

- **Smart Materials**: Emerging smart materials have the potential to change the landscape of orthodontics. For example, materials that can respond to temperature changes or light could allow aligners to gradually adjust their properties, enhancing treatment efficacy.

Example: Aligners made from smart materials might adapt their stiffness based on the temperature of the mouth, providing optimal force for tooth movement.

2. AI and Machine Learning in Treatment Planning

AI-Driven Treatment Planning

- **Predictive Analytics**: AI algorithms analyze vast amounts of data from previous cases to predict treatment outcomes with high accuracy. This predictive capability allows for more precise planning of tooth movements and adjustments.

- **Automated Adjustments**: AI can automate the creation of treatment plans by analyzing digital scans and X-rays. This reduces the time required for manual planning and minimizes human error.

Example: An orthodontist uses an AI-driven platform to input a patient's dental scans. The AI generates a comprehensive treatment plan with estimated timelines and expected outcomes, streamlining the planning process.

Machine Learning Algorithms

- **Continuous Improvement**: Machine learning algorithms continuously improve by learning from new data and treatment outcomes. This leads to more refined and effective treatment plans over time.

- **Personalized Treatment Plans**: Machine learning models can tailor treatment plans based on individual patient characteristics, such as the specific alignment issues and dental anatomy, providing a more personalized approach.

Example: A machine learning algorithm analyzes data from thousands of cases to create a customized aligner plan that accounts for the patient's unique dental structure and treatment needs.

3. The Future of Teledentistry and At-Home Aligner Systems

Teledentistry

- **Remote Consultations**: Teledentistry allows for virtual consultations between patients and orthodontists. Patients can receive initial assessments, follow-up care, and even treatment adjustments without needing to visit the office in person.

- **Real-Time Monitoring**: With the use of digital tools and remote monitoring devices, orthodontists can track treatment progress in real-time and make timely adjustments to the aligners if needed.

Example: A patient using a teledentistry platform submits photos and videos of their aligners and teeth. The orthodontist reviews the data and provides remote guidance on adjustments.

At-Home Aligner Systems

- **Direct-to-Consumer Models**: At-home aligner systems, offered by companies like Smile Direct Club, allow patients to undergo treatment without in-office visits. Patients receive a kit to take impressions of their teeth and receive aligners through mail.

- **Convenience and Accessibility**: These systems offer a convenient and cost-effective alternative to traditional orthodontic care, making clear aligners more accessible to a broader audience.

Example: A patient opts for an at-home aligner system and uses a DIY impression kit to start treatment. They receive aligners and follow instructions remotely, with periodic virtual check-ins.

4. Customization and Personalization in Orthodontic Care

Custom Aligners

- **Individualized Fit**: Custom aligners are designed based on detailed 3D scans of the patient's teeth. This customization ensures a precise fit and effective movement of teeth.

- **Tailored Treatment Plans**: Each aligner is crafted to address specific dental issues, such as spacing, crowding, or bite correction, based on the patient's unique needs.

Example: A patient with complex alignment issues receives a series of custom-made aligners designed to address each specific issue in a step-by-step approach.

Personalized Care

- **Adaptive Treatments**: Personalization extends beyond aligner design to include adaptive treatment plans. Orthodontists adjust treatment based on real-time feedback and progress.

- **Patient Preferences**: Personalization also involves accommodating patient preferences, such as aligner wear schedules and adjustments, to enhance comfort and adherence to treatment.

Example: A patient prefers to wear aligners only during the evenings. The orthodontist adjusts the treatment plan accordingly to ensure effective tooth movement while accommodating the patient's schedule.

Summary

Technological innovations in clear aligners have significantly advanced the field of orthodontics. Advances in 3D printing and material science have improved the precision, durability, and comfort of aligners. AI and machine learning are enhancing treatment planning by providing predictive analytics and personalized plans. The rise of teledentistry and at-home aligner systems is making orthodontic care more accessible and convenient. Finally, customization and personalization in orthodontic care ensure that treatments are tailored to individual patient needs, improving overall outcomes and satisfaction.

Chapter 9

Clear Aligners vs. Traditional Braces

Orthodontic treatment has evolved significantly over the years, with clear aligners emerging as a modern alternative to traditional metal braces. This chapter delves into a comprehensive comparison between clear aligners and traditional braces, covering aspects such as effectiveness, cost, patient satisfaction, treatment timelines, predictability, ideal patient profiles, and the impact on lifestyle and aesthetics. We will explore these elements from historical perspectives to future trends in orthodontic care.

1. Historical Overview of Orthodontic Treatments

Early Orthodontics

- **Ancient Techniques**: The history of orthodontics dates back to ancient civilizations. Archaeological evidence suggests that early orthodontic techniques involved rudimentary metal bands and wires. Ancient Egyptians and Greeks used simple methods to correct dental misalignments.

- **18th and 19th Centuries**: The development of orthodontics as a formal field began in the 18th and 19th centuries. Pierre Fauchard, a French dentist, is often credited with pioneering orthodontic practices, including the use of metal bands and appliances. Edward Angle, an American orthodontist, further advanced the field with the introduction of the Angle classification system and the development of fixed appliances.

Introduction of Modern Appliances

- **1960s and 1970s**: The late 20th century saw the advent of modern orthodontic appliances. Metal braces became widely used, characterized by their brackets and archwires, which provided effective correction for a range of malocclusions. These braces, though effective, were often perceived as bulky and aesthetically unappealing.

Emergence of Clear Aligners

- **Late 1990s**: The late 1990s marked the introduction of clear aligners, pioneered by Align Technology. The concept of clear aligners revolutionized orthodontics by offering a more discreet and comfortable alternative to traditional braces. The initial clear aligner systems were based on innovative computer modeling and 3D printing technology, paving the way for modern orthodontics.

2. Comparing Effectiveness

Clear Aligners

- **Effectiveness for Mild to Moderate Cases**: Clear aligners are highly effective for treating mild to moderate dental misalignments, including spacing, crowding, and some bite issues. They use a series of custom-made aligners to gradually move teeth into the desired position.

- **Limitations**: For severe malocclusions or complex orthodontic issues, clear aligners may be less effective compared to traditional braces. Cases involving significant bite problems, complex rotations, or vertical discrepancies might require adjunctive treatments or are better addressed with traditional braces.

Traditional Braces

- **Versatility and Effectiveness**: Traditional braces are effective for a wide range of orthodontic problems, including severe crowding, significant bite issues, and complex malocclusions. The fixed nature of braces allows for precise control of tooth movements and can address more challenging cases.

- **Braces Mechanics**: Braces use brackets bonded to each tooth and an archwire to apply continuous pressure, which gradually shifts teeth into the correct position. This method provides consistent and reliable results for complex cases.

Comparative Example: A patient with severe crowding may achieve better results with traditional braces due to their ability to exert more precise and consistent forces on the teeth compared to clear aligners.

3. Cost Considerations

Clear Aligners

- **Initial Cost**: Clear aligners generally have a higher initial cost compared to traditional braces. This cost reflects the advanced technology and customization involved in creating and manufacturing the aligners.

- **Long-Term Costs**: The overall cost of clear aligner treatment can vary based on the complexity of the case and the number of aligners required. Additional expenses may include follow-up visits and potential replacement aligners if lost or damaged.

Traditional Braces

- **Initial Cost**: Traditional braces typically have a lower initial cost compared to clear aligners. The cost includes the braces, bonding materials, and archwires.

- **Long-Term Costs**: The long-term cost of traditional braces is often lower due to fewer additional expenses. However, patients may need to account for occasional adjustments and repairs.

Cost Example: A comprehensive treatment plan for clear aligners may range from $4,000 to $8,000, while traditional braces may cost between $3,000 and $7,000, depending on the complexity and geographic location.

4. Patient Satisfaction

Clear Aligners

- **Comfort and Convenience**: Patients often report higher

satisfaction with clear aligners due to their comfort and convenience. Aligners are removable, allowing for easier maintenance of oral hygiene and flexibility in eating.

- **Aesthetic Appeal**: The invisibility of clear aligners is a significant factor in patient satisfaction. Many patients prefer clear aligners over traditional braces for their discreet appearance.

Traditional Braces

- **Effectiveness and Control**: Patients with traditional braces may experience a higher level of satisfaction in cases where precise control over tooth movement is essential. The fixed nature of braces provides consistent and predictable results.

- **Adjustments and Maintenance**: While traditional braces can be less comfortable due to the brackets and wires, patients may appreciate the durability and effectiveness in correcting more complex orthodontic issues.

Patient Satisfaction Example: A patient undergoing treatment for mild alignment issues may prefer clear aligners for their comfort and aesthetics, while a patient with severe malocclusions may be more satisfied with traditional braces due to their effectiveness in addressing complex problems.

5. Treatment Timelines and Predictability

Clear Aligners

- **Treatment Duration**: Clear aligner treatment typically ranges from 6 to 18 months, depending on the complexity of the case. The duration may be shorter for mild cases and longer for more complex issues.

- **Predictability**: Clear aligners offer a high degree of predictability due to the use of digital treatment planning and 3D modeling. However, adjustments may be needed if treatment progress does not align with initial projections.

Traditional Braces

• **Treatment Duration**: Treatment with traditional braces usually lasts between 18 to 36 months. The duration depends on the severity of the malocclusion and the individual's response to treatment.

• **Predictability**: Traditional braces provide consistent and predictable results due to the fixed nature of the appliance. Adjustments and modifications can be made during regular visits to ensure continued progress.

Example: A patient with mild crowding might complete treatment with clear aligners in 8 months, while a patient with severe crowding may need traditional braces for up to 24 months.

6. Ideal Patient Profiles for Each Option

Clear Aligners

• **Ideal Candidates**: Clear aligners are best suited for individuals with mild to moderate dental misalignments, such as slight crowding, spacing, or minor bite issues. They are also ideal for adults and teens seeking a discreet treatment option.

• **Patient Compliance**: Patients must be disciplined in wearing aligners for the recommended 20-22 hours per day to achieve optimal results. Non-compliance can lead to extended treatment times and less predictable outcomes.

Traditional Braces

• **Ideal Candidates**: Traditional braces are ideal for patients with more complex orthodontic issues, such as severe crowding, significant bite problems, or substantial malocclusions. They are also effective for younger patients who may not be as compliant with removable appliances.

• **Adaptability**: Traditional braces are suitable for patients who need precise and reliable control over tooth movements, including those with complex cases or those requiring multiple phases of treatment.

Patient Profile Example: A teenager with a complex malocclusion might benefit more from traditional braces, while an adult with minor spacing issues may prefer clear aligners for their discreet nature.

7. Impact on Lifestyle and Aesthetics

Clear Aligners

- **Lifestyle Benefits**: Clear aligners offer significant lifestyle benefits, including the ability to remove the aligners for eating and oral hygiene. This flexibility allows patients to maintain their normal diet and brushing routine without restrictions.

- **Aesthetic Impact**: The nearly invisible nature of clear aligners enhances patient comfort and confidence, particularly for adults and professionals concerned about the appearance of traditional braces.

Traditional Braces

- **Lifestyle Considerations**: Traditional braces can impact lifestyle by requiring dietary modifications and careful oral hygiene practices to avoid damage to the brackets and wires. Patients may need to avoid sticky or hard foods that could damage the braces.

- **Aesthetic Impact**: The visibility of traditional braces can affect aesthetics and self-esteem, especially for adults and teenagers who may feel self-conscious about their appearance during treatment.

Lifestyle and Aesthetic Example: A professional seeking a discreet treatment option might prefer clear aligners to avoid the visual impact of traditional braces, while a patient needing extensive correction may prioritize effectiveness over aesthetics.

8. Future Trends and Innovations

Technological Advancements

- **Improved Materials**: Future developments in aligner materials may lead to even greater comfort, durability, and effectiveness. Advances in material science could enhance the performance of clear aligners in treating complex cases.

- **Enhanced Digital Planning**: Continued advancements in digital technology, including AI and machine learning, will further refine treatment planning and predictability for both clear aligners and traditional braces.

Integration of Teledentistry

- **Remote Monitoring**: The integration of teledentistry in orthodontic care will likely expand, allowing for more frequent and convenient remote monitoring of treatment progress. This will benefit both clear aligner and traditional brace patients by enhancing the efficiency of care.

Customization and Personalization

- **Tailored Treatments**: Future orthodontic treatments will increasingly focus on customization and personalization, providing patients with treatment plans that are specifically designed to address their unique dental needs and preferences.

Future Example: An orthodontic practice may offer a hybrid treatment approach that combines clear aligners with advanced digital tools and teledentistry to provide a more comprehensive and personalized orthodontic experience.

Summary

The comparison between clear aligners and traditional braces highlights the strengths and limitations of each treatment option. Clear aligners offer advantages in terms of aesthetics, comfort, and convenience but may not be suitable for all cases. Traditional braces provide effective solutions for a wide range of orthodontic issues, particularly complex cases, but come with considerations related to aesthetics and lifestyle impact. As orthodontic technology continues to evolve, both treatment options are likely to benefit from advancements in materials, digital planning, and personalization, shaping the future of orthodontic care.

Table summarizing the key aspects of clear aligners versus traditional braces:

Aspect	Clear Aligners	Traditional Braces
Effectiveness	Effective for mild to moderate cases. Less effective for severe malocclusions and complex issues.	Highly effective for a wide range of cases, including severe malocclusions and complex issues.
Cost	Typically higher initial cost ($4,000 - $8,000). May have additional expenses for follow-up visits and replacements.	Generally lower initial cost ($3,000 - $7,000). Fewer additional costs.
Patient Satisfaction	High satisfaction due to comfort, convenience, and aesthetics. Removable for easy oral hygiene.	Satisfaction depends on effectiveness and control. Less comfort and aesthetics compared to aligners.
Treatment Duration	Usually 6 to 18 months, depending on complexity. Shorter for mild cases, longer for complex issues.	Typically 18 to 36 months. Duration varies with complexity and individual response.
Predictability	High predictability with digital planning and 3D modeling. Adjustments may be needed if progress deviates.	Consistent and predictable results due to fixed appliances and regular adjustments.
Ideal Patient Profile	Best for individuals with mild to moderate	Ideal for those with complex or severe

	misalignments. Ideal for adults and teens seeking discreet treatment.	orthodontic issues. Suitable for younger patients and those needing precise control.
Lifestyle Impact	Minimal lifestyle changes required. Aligners are removable, allowing for normal eating and oral hygiene.	Requires dietary modifications (avoiding sticky or hard foods). Brushing and flossing are more challenging.
Aesthetic Impact	Nearly invisible, offering a discreet treatment option. Preferred by adults and professionals.	Visible and noticeable, which can impact self-esteem and appearance, particularly for adults.
Comfort	Generally more comfortable. No metal brackets or wires. Aligners can cause temporary discomfort.	Can cause discomfort due to brackets and wires. Adjustments may lead to soreness and irritation.
Technology	Utilizes advanced 3D printing, digital modeling, and material science.	Traditional braces use brackets and wires with less advanced technology.
Compliance	Requires disciplined adherence to wearing aligners 20-22 hours per day. Non-compliance can extend treatment time.	Fixed nature ensures constant treatment pressure. No need for patient compliance in wearing.
Maintenance	Easier to maintain oral hygiene. Aligners can be removed for brushing and flossing.	Requires meticulous oral hygiene to avoid plaque buildup around brackets and wires.
Adaptability	Customizable based on patient scans. Suitable for gradual adjustments.	Less customizable. Adjustments are made during office visits.

Future Trends	Advances in materials and digital planning. Integration with teledentistry for remote monitoring.	Continued use of fixed appliances with potential enhancements in materials and digital technology.

Chapter 10

The Business of Clear Aligners

The business landscape for clear aligners has experienced transformative changes, largely influenced by rapid technological advancements, evolving consumer preferences, and competitive market dynamics. This chapter provides an in-depth exploration of these elements, beginning with the burgeoning market for clear aligners and examining the industry trends shaping their growth.

The clear aligner market has witnessed exponential growth over recent years, driven by an increasing demand for discreet orthodontic solutions. As patients seek more aesthetically pleasing and comfortable alternatives to traditional metal braces, clear aligners have become a popular choice. Market research indicates a significant rise in the number of patients opting for clear aligners, reflecting their growing acceptance among diverse demographic groups, including adults and teenagers. This surge in popularity is supported by advancements in aligner technology, which have enhanced treatment efficacy and patient experience.

1. The Growing Market and Industry Trends

Market Growth

- **Expanding Demand**: The clear aligner market has experienced rapid growth due to increasing awareness of orthodontic options and demand for aesthetically pleasing solutions. Factors contributing to this growth include the rising prevalence of dental misalignments, a growing emphasis on cosmetic dentistry, and advancements in aligner technology.

- **Market Size**: The global clear aligner market was valued at approximately $3.5 billion in 2020 and is projected to reach around $6.5 billion by 2025, with a compound annual growth rate (CAGR) of about

12%. This growth reflects both an expanding patient base and advancements in aligner technology.

Industry Trends

• **Technological Innovations**: Continued advancements in 3D printing, digital modeling, and material science are driving innovations in clear aligner technology. These advancements enhance the precision, comfort, and effectiveness of aligners.

• **Increased Adoption**: Clear aligners are becoming increasingly popular among adults and teens, as they offer a discreet and convenient orthodontic solution. The rise in direct-to-consumer (DTC) aligner companies has further fueled this trend by making aligners more accessible.

Example: The entry of new players into the market, such as Smile Direct Club and Candid, has intensified competition and led to innovations in treatment options and pricing structures.

2. Marketing Strategies and Consumer Outreach

Effective Marketing Strategies

• **Digital Marketing**: Companies utilize digital marketing strategies, including social media advertising, influencer partnerships, and targeted online ads, to reach potential customers. Social media platforms like Instagram and TikTok are effective in showcasing treatment results and engaging with a younger audience.

• **Educational Content**: Providing educational content about clear aligners, including blogs, videos, and webinars, helps build trust and informs potential patients about the benefits and process of aligner therapy.

Consumer Outreach

• **Customer Reviews and Testimonials**: Positive reviews and testimonials play a crucial role in consumer decision-making. Aligners companies often feature patient success stories and before-and-after photos to build credibility and attract new clients.

• **Virtual Consultations**: Many aligner companies offer virtual consultations, allowing potential patients to receive initial evaluations and treatment plans from the comfort of their homes. This approach enhances accessibility and convenience.

Example: Invisalign's successful use of social media campaigns and partnerships with influencers has significantly boosted brand visibility and consumer engagement.

3. Regulatory Considerations and Ethical Concerns

Regulatory Framework

• **FDA and CE Approval**: Clear aligner manufacturers must comply with regulatory standards such as FDA approval in the United States and CE marking in Europe. These approvals ensure that aligners meet safety and effectiveness criteria.

• **Quality Control**: Regulatory bodies require strict quality control measures to ensure the safety and efficacy of aligners. Manufacturers must adhere to guidelines for material quality, manufacturing processes, and clinical testing.

Ethical Concerns

• **Direct-to-Consumer Risks**: DTC aligner companies have faced criticism for bypassing in-person evaluations by orthodontists. This approach can pose risks if patients with complex orthodontic needs are not properly assessed by professionals.

• **Transparency**: Ethical concerns include ensuring transparency in pricing, treatment options, and potential outcomes. Clear aligner companies must provide accurate information to avoid misleading claims and ensure informed patient decisions.

Example: Concerns about the quality of care provided by DTC aligner companies have led to increased scrutiny and calls for stricter regulations and oversight.

4. Role of General Dentists vs. Orthodontists in Aligner Therapy

General Dentists

- **Role**: General dentists can prescribe and oversee clear aligner treatments for patients with mild to moderate orthodontic issues. They may work in collaboration with orthodontists for more complex cases.

- **Training and Expertise**: General dentists need to undergo additional training to provide clear aligner therapy effectively. Many opt for certification programs and continuing education to stay updated on aligner technologies and treatment techniques.

Orthodontists

- **Role**: Orthodontists are specialized in diagnosing and treating a wide range of orthodontic issues, including complex cases. They often handle more challenging aligner cases and provide comprehensive treatment planning and monitoring.

- **Expertise**: Orthodontists have advanced training in orthodontics and are well-equipped to handle intricate cases that may not be suitable for general dentists. They also use their expertise to ensure precise treatment outcomes and address any complications that may arise.

Example: An orthodontist might be consulted for a patient with severe bite issues, while a general dentist may handle a patient seeking clear aligners for mild crowding.

Chapter 11

The Future of Clear Aligners

As the orthodontic industry continues to evolve, clear aligners are poised to play an increasingly prominent role. This chapter explores upcoming technologies, emerging brands, competitive landscape, and future trends in personalized orthodontics, with a focus on potential improvements in patient experience and outcomes.

1. Upcoming Technologies and Industry Shifts

Advancements in Materials

- **New Materials**: Research into advanced materials for clear aligners aims to improve durability, flexibility, and comfort. Innovations in material science could lead to aligners that are even less noticeable and more effective.

- **Smart Aligners**: Development of smart aligners equipped with sensors and data tracking capabilities could provide real-time monitoring of treatment progress and patient compliance.

Integration of AI and Machine Learning

- **Treatment Planning**: AI and machine learning are expected to enhance treatment planning by analyzing large datasets to predict outcomes and optimize aligner design. These technologies will improve the precision and efficiency of treatment.

- **Predictive Analytics**: AI-driven predictive analytics will help in customizing treatment plans and anticipating potential complications, leading to more tailored and effective orthodontic care.

Example: Companies like Align Technology are investing in AI-driven treatment planning tools to enhance the accuracy and predictability of clear aligner treatments.

2. Emerging Brands and Competitive Landscape

New Market Entrants

- **Innovative Companies**: New brands and startups are entering the clear aligner market, bringing innovative approaches and competitive pricing. These companies often leverage advanced technology and direct-to-consumer models to differentiate themselves.

- **Increased Competition**: The growing number of players in the market is leading to increased competition, which drives innovation and provides patients with more options.

Competitive Strategies

- **Differentiation**: Emerging brands are focusing on differentiating themselves through unique features, such as customizable aligners, enhanced comfort, and flexible treatment options. They also emphasize affordability and accessibility.

- **Partnerships and Collaborations**: Collaboration between aligner companies and dental professionals is becoming more common, with partnerships aimed at improving patient care and expanding market reach.

Example: New entrants like Candid and Byte are gaining traction by offering affordable clear aligner solutions and leveraging online platforms for patient engagement.

3. Future Trends in Personalized Orthodontics

Customization and Personalization

- **Tailored Treatments**: Future trends will emphasize highly personalized orthodontic care, with treatments customized to individual patient needs and preferences. Advances in digital technology will enable more precise and personalized treatment plans.

- **Patient-Centered Care**: Personalized care will focus on enhancing patient experience, addressing specific concerns, and accommodating lifestyle preferences. This approach aims to improve patient satisfaction and treatment outcomes.

Integration with Teledentistry

• **Remote Monitoring**: The integration of teledentistry with clear aligner therapy will enable remote monitoring of treatment progress, providing patients with greater convenience and reducing the need for in-person visits.

• **Virtual Consultations**: Continued growth in virtual consultations will make orthodontic care more accessible, particularly for patients in remote or underserved areas.

Example: Platforms that offer virtual consultations and remote monitoring, combined with personalized aligner designs, will become increasingly prevalent, enhancing the overall patient experience.

4. Potential Improvements in Patient Experience and Outcomes

Enhanced Comfort and Convenience

• **Improved Aligner Design**: Future advancements in aligner design will focus on enhancing comfort, reducing treatment time, and minimizing discomfort. Innovations in materials and technology will contribute to a more pleasant treatment experience.

• **Streamlined Processes**: The use of advanced technology will streamline the treatment process, making it more efficient and convenient for patients. This includes faster scanning, quicker aligner production, and more accurate treatment planning.

Better Treatment Outcomes

• **Predictive Modeling**: Improved predictive modeling and data analysis will lead to more accurate treatment outcomes and reduced risk of complications. Enhanced digital tools will enable orthodontists to fine-tune treatment plans and achieve optimal results.

- **Patient Feedback Integration**: Incorporating patient feedback into treatment planning and adjustments will further refine and personalize orthodontic care, leading to improved patient satisfaction and results.

Example: Advanced predictive modeling tools that analyze patient data in real-time will enhance the accuracy of treatment plans and contribute to better overall outcomes.

Summary

The business of clear aligners is rapidly evolving, driven by technological advancements, shifting consumer preferences, and increasing competition. As the industry progresses, innovations in materials, digital planning, and patient-centered care will shape the future of clear aligner therapy. Emerging brands and technological advancements will continue to enhance the patient experience, while regulatory considerations and ethical concerns will play a crucial role in ensuring safe and effective orthodontic care.

Conclusion: The Clear Aligner Revolution

The clear aligner revolution has significantly transformed orthodontic care, making it more accessible, comfortable, and aesthetically pleasing. As this technology continues to evolve, it's essential to understand the key points of clear aligners, their growing popularity, and how to choose the right orthodontic treatment for individual needs. This conclusion encapsulates the essence of clear aligners and provides insights into their impact on modern orthodontics.

Recap of Key Points

1. Historical Context

- **Evolution of Orthodontics**: Traditional orthodontic treatments began with metal braces and gradually evolved to include more sophisticated and discreet options. The introduction of clear aligners marked a significant milestone in this evolution, offering patients a less noticeable and more comfortable alternative to traditional braces.

2. Clear Aligner Technology

- **Science and Mechanics**: Clear aligners use advanced technology, including 3D scanning and digital modeling, to create customized treatment plans. Aligners are made from high-quality, flexible materials designed to gradually shift teeth into their desired positions.

- **Process and Effectiveness**: The treatment process involves a series of aligners, each designed to move teeth incrementally. Clear aligners are effective for various orthodontic issues, particularly mild to moderate cases, and offer a high degree of predictability due to digital planning.

3. Types of Clear Aligners

- **Brands and Technologies**: Major brands such as Invisalign, ClearCorrect, and Smile Direct Club offer different technologies and features. In-office aligners provide more personalized care, while direct-to-consumer aligners offer affordability and convenience but may lack professional oversight.

4. Advantages

- **Aesthetics and Comfort**: Clear aligners are virtually invisible, providing a discreet treatment option. They are also removable, allowing for better oral hygiene and comfort compared to traditional braces.

- **Predictability and Convenience**: Digital planning and 3D modeling enhance the accuracy of treatment outcomes. Aligners are designed to fit seamlessly into patients' lifestyles, requiring fewer office visits and allowing for easier maintenance.

5. Limitations and Challenges

- **Suitability**: Clear aligners are not ideal for all cases, particularly those involving severe malocclusions or complex orthodontic issues.

Compliance and patient discipline are crucial for achieving desired results.

- **Cost and Accessibility**: The cost of clear aligners can be higher than traditional braces, and some patients may face challenges in accessing or affording treatment.

6. Patient Experience

- **Journey and Care**: The patient journey with clear aligners involves initial consultations, understanding the treatment timeline, and managing any discomfort or challenges. The retention phase is critical for maintaining results, and patients must adhere to retainer protocols post-treatment.

7. Clinical Applications

- **Case Studies**: Clear aligners have been successfully used to address a range of orthodontic issues, including mild crowding, spacing, overbite, and underbite corrections. Case studies highlight the effectiveness and versatility of clear aligners in various clinical scenarios.

8. Technological Innovations

- **Future Trends**: Advances in 3D printing, AI, and teledentistry are shaping the future of clear aligners. Innovations are expected to enhance treatment precision, comfort, and overall patient experience.

9. Comparative Analysis

- **Clear Aligners vs. Traditional Braces**: Clear aligners offer aesthetic and comfort advantages, while traditional braces are effective for complex cases. The choice between aligners and braces depends on individual needs, preferences, and treatment goals.

10. The Business Landscape

- **Market Dynamics**: The clear aligner market is growing rapidly, driven by technological advancements and increased consumer demand. Marketing strategies, regulatory considerations, and the roles of dental professionals play significant roles in shaping the industry.

The Growing Popularity and Mainstream Acceptance

Clear aligners have gained widespread acceptance among patients seeking discreet and convenient orthodontic solutions. Their popularity is driven by several factors:

- **Aesthetic Appeal**: The nearly invisible nature of clear aligners appeals to individuals who prefer a less noticeable treatment option.

- **Convenience**: Removable aligners offer greater flexibility and ease of maintenance compared to traditional braces.

- **Technological Advancements**: Continued innovations in aligner technology enhance treatment outcomes and patient satisfaction.

Clear aligners are becoming a mainstream choice for orthodontic treatment, with increasing numbers of patients opting for this modern solution. The growth of direct-to-consumer aligner companies has further contributed to the mainstream acceptance of clear aligners, making them more accessible to a broader audience.

Final Thoughts on Choosing the Right Orthodontic Treatment

Choosing the right orthodontic treatment involves considering various factors, including:

- **Treatment Goals**: Assessing the specific orthodontic issues and desired outcomes will help determine the most suitable treatment option. Clear aligners are ideal for mild to moderate cases, while traditional braces may be necessary for more complex issues.

- **Patient Preferences**: Aesthetic preferences, comfort, and lifestyle considerations play a crucial role in selecting the appropriate treatment. Clear aligners offer a discreet and comfortable option, while traditional braces provide a tried-and-true solution for complex cases.

- **Professional Consultation**: Consulting with a dental professional, such as an orthodontist or general dentist, is essential for evaluating treatment options and developing a personalized plan. Professional guidance ensures that patients make informed decisions based on their unique needs and circumstances. Ultimately, the choice between clear aligners and traditional braces should be based on a comprehensive assessment of individual needs, treatment goals, and personal preferences. Both options offer valuable benefits, and advancements in orthodontic technology will continue to shape the future of dental care.

Appendix

Glossary of Key Terms

Aligners:

Aligners are custom-made, clear plastic trays designed to gently shift teeth into their proper alignment. They are a popular alternative to traditional metal braces due to their discreet appearance and removable nature. Each aligner is designed to make incremental adjustments to the teeth over time. Patients typically wear each set of aligners for a few weeks before progressing to the next set in the series, which is tailored to continue the alignment process. Aligners are made from medical-grade plastic and are created using advanced 3D technology to ensure a precise fit and effective treatment.

3D Scanning:

3D scanning is a cutting-edge technology used in orthodontics to create detailed digital models of a patient's teeth, gums, and mouth. This process involves using a specialized scanner to capture precise measurements and images, which are then used to construct a virtual 3D representation of the patient's oral anatomy. The digital model allows orthodontists to plan and simulate the treatment process accurately, design custom aligners, and visualize the projected results before treatment begins. 3D scanning enhances the accuracy of aligner fitting and treatment outcomes.

Digital Modeling:

Digital modeling refers to the process of creating a virtual, three-dimensional representation of a patient's teeth and bite using computer software. This model is generated from the data obtained through 3D scanning and is used to plan and simulate orthodontic treatment. Digital modeling allows orthodontists to design aligners with precise measurements and predict the movement of teeth throughout the treatment. It also facilitates the creation of treatment simulations that help both the patient and the orthodontist visualize the anticipated results and make informed decisions about the treatment plan.

Malocclusion:

Malocclusion is a term used to describe a misalignment of the teeth and bite. It occurs when the teeth do not fit together correctly, which can lead to various dental issues such as difficulty chewing, speech problems, and increased risk of dental decay or gum disease. Malocclusion can manifest in different forms, including overcrowding, spacing issues, overbites, underbites, and crossbites. The severity of malocclusion can vary from mild to severe, and it often requires orthodontic intervention to correct the alignment and improve overall oral health and function.

Retention Phase:

The retention phase is the final stage of orthodontic treatment, following the active phase where teeth are aligned using braces or clear aligners. During this phase, retainers are used to maintain the corrected position of the teeth and prevent them from shifting back to their original positions. Retainers can be removable or fixed, and their use is crucial for ensuring long-term treatment success. The duration of the retention phase varies depending on individual needs and the specific orthodontic issues addressed. Consistent use of retainers as prescribed by the orthodontist is essential for preserving the results achieved during treatment.

Clear Aligners:

Clear aligners are a modern orthodontic treatment method that uses a series of transparent, removable trays to gradually move teeth into their ideal positions. Unlike traditional braces, clear aligners are virtually invisible, making them a popular choice for patients seeking a more discreet treatment option. The aligners are custom-made from high-quality plastic materials and are designed based on digital impressions and treatment planning. Clear aligners offer a comfortable and convenient alternative to metal braces, with the added benefit of being removable for eating, drinking, and oral hygiene.

Orthodontic Treatment Plan:

An orthodontic treatment plan is a comprehensive strategy developed by an orthodontist to address and correct specific dental and orthodontic issues. The plan includes detailed information about the goals of treatment, the methods and appliances to be used (such as clear aligners or braces), the estimated duration of treatment, and the steps involved in achieving the desired outcomes. The treatment plan is personalized based on the patient's unique needs and is created using diagnostic tools such as X-rays, 3D scans, and digital models.

Interproximal Reduction (IPR):

Interproximal reduction (IPR) is a technique used in orthodontics to create space between teeth by selectively removing small amounts of enamel from the interproximal areas (the surfaces between adjacent teeth). This procedure is often used in conjunction with clear aligner treatment to address issues such as mild overcrowding or to achieve more precise tooth movements. IPR is a conservative approach that helps improve the fit and alignment of the teeth without the need for more invasive procedures.

Bite Alignment:

Bite alignment refers to the proper relationship between the upper and lower teeth when the mouth is closed. Achieving correct bite alignment is essential for optimal dental function and overall oral health. Common bite issues include overbites, underbites, crossbites, and open bites. Clear aligners and other orthodontic treatments are designed to correct these bite issues by gradually repositioning the teeth and improving the alignment of the dental arches.

Compliance:

Compliance in orthodontics refers to the patient's adherence to the prescribed treatment plan and instructions provided by the orthodontist. This includes wearing aligners for the recommended number of hours each day, following oral hygiene guidelines, attending scheduled appointments, and using retainers as directed after treatment. High compliance is critical for achieving successful treatment outcomes with clear aligners and ensuring that the teeth remain in their corrected positions.

Retainers:

Retainers are orthodontic appliances used to maintain the results achieved during the active phase of orthodontic treatment. They help prevent teeth from shifting back to their original positions and ensure that the alignment achieved with braces or clear aligners is preserved. Retainers can be removable or fixed, and they are typically worn for a specified period following the completion of active treatment. The type and duration of retainer use vary depending on the individual's treatment plan and orthodontic needs.

Orthodontic Appliances:

Orthodontic appliances are devices used to correct misalignments and bite issues in the teeth and jaws. They include a variety of tools, such as braces, clear aligners, retainers, and expanders. Each type of appliance serves a specific purpose and is selected based on the patient's orthodontic needs. Orthodontic appliances work by applying gentle pressure to the teeth and jaws to achieve gradual and controlled movements.

Tooth Movement:

Tooth movement refers to the gradual shifting of teeth into new positions as part of orthodontic treatment. This process is achieved through the application of controlled forces using appliances such as clear aligners or braces. The movement of teeth is guided by the treatment plan, which takes into account the patient's specific orthodontic issues and goals. Effective tooth movement requires precise planning and consistent use of the prescribed orthodontic appliances.

Aligner Tray:

An aligner tray is a custom-made, transparent plastic device used in clear aligner therapy to move teeth into their desired positions. Each tray is designed to fit snugly over the patient's teeth and apply gentle, consistent pressure to guide tooth movement. Aligners are worn in a sequence, with each tray representing a stage in the treatment process. The number of trays required depends on the complexity of the case and the treatment plan.

Orthodontic Evaluation:

An orthodontic evaluation is a comprehensive assessment conducted by an orthodontist to diagnose and determine the appropriate treatment for dental and orthodontic issues. The evaluation includes a review of the patient's dental history, a physical examination of the teeth and jaws, and the use of diagnostic tools such as X-rays, 3D scans, and digital impressions. The results of the evaluation are used to develop a personalized treatment plan and address any concerns or questions the patient may have.

Digital Impressions:

Digital impressions are a modern method of capturing accurate, three-dimensional images of a patient's teeth and oral structures. This technique replaces traditional mold impressions with a digital scanner that records detailed images of the teeth and gums. Digital impressions are used to create precise models for treatment planning, aligner fabrication, and other orthodontic procedures. They offer several advantages, including improved accuracy, faster results, and greater patient comfort.

Orthodontic Consultation:

An orthodontic consultation is an initial meeting between a patient and an orthodontist to discuss potential treatment options for addressing dental and orthodontic issues. During the consultation, the orthodontist evaluates the patient's oral health, discusses treatment goals, and provides information about available treatment methods, such as clear aligners or braces. The consultation is an opportunity for patients to ask questions, understand their treatment options, and make informed decisions about their orthodontic care.

Custom Aligners:

Custom aligners are individualized clear trays designed specifically for each patient based on their unique dental needs and treatment goals. Using digital impressions and 3D modeling, orthodontists create aligners that fit precisely over the patient's teeth and apply targeted pressure to achieve desired tooth movements. Custom aligners are essential for effective orthodontic treatment, ensuring that each stage of the treatment plan is tailored to the patient's specific requirements.

Treatment Duration:

Treatment duration refers to the total length of time required to complete orthodontic treatment and achieve the desired results. For clear aligners, treatment duration varies based on factors such as the complexity of the case, the degree of tooth movement needed, and the patient's compliance with the treatment plan. On average, clear aligner treatments take between 6 to 18 months, but this can vary from patient to patient.

Orthodontic Diagnosis:

Orthodontic diagnosis involves identifying and analyzing dental and skeletal issues that require correction through orthodontic treatment. The diagnosis is based on a combination of clinical examinations, diagnostic imaging, and patient history. Accurate diagnosis is crucial for developing an effective treatment plan and selecting the appropriate orthodontic appliances to address the patient's specific needs.

Patient Compliance:

Patient compliance refers to the extent to which a patient follows the orthodontist's instructions and treatment plan. High compliance is critical for the success of orthodontic treatment, particularly with clear aligners, which require consistent wear to achieve the desired tooth movements. Non-compliance can lead to extended treatment times, suboptimal results, and the need for additional adjustments or interventions.

Treatment Planning:

Treatment planning is the process of developing a detailed strategy for orthodontic treatment based on the patient's specific dental and orthodontic needs. This process involves creating a comprehensive plan that outlines the goals of treatment, the methods and appliances to be used, the estimated duration, and the steps required to achieve the desired outcomes. Treatment planning is informed by diagnostic information, including digital impressions, 3D scans, and clinical evaluations.

Aligner Attachments:

Aligner attachments are small, tooth-colored bumps or buttons placed on the teeth to enhance the effectiveness of clear aligners. These attachments help the aligners grip and apply pressure to specific areas of the teeth, facilitating more complex movements that may not be achievable with aligners alone. Attachments are used as part of the treatment plan to address specific orthodontic issues and achieve more precise tooth movements.

Space Maintainers:

Space maintainers are devices used to hold open space in the dental arch after the premature loss of a primary tooth. They are used to ensure that the permanent teeth have enough room to emerge and align properly. Space maintainers are commonly used in pediatric orthodontics and may be needed if a child loses a primary tooth before the permanent tooth is ready to come in.

Functional Appliances:

Functional appliances are orthodontic devices designed to modify the growth and development of the jaws and improve the relationship between the upper and lower teeth. They are often used in growing children and adolescents to address issues such as overbites, underbites, and crossbites. Functional appliances work by applying forces to the teeth and jaws to guide their development and correct alignment.

Orthodontic Retainer Types:

Orthodontic retainers come in various types, including removable and fixed retainers. Removable retainers are designed to be taken out for eating and oral hygiene, while fixed retainers are bonded to the teeth and remain in place permanently. The type of retainer used depends on the patient's treatment plan and the specific needs for maintaining the results achieved with braces or clear aligners.

Aligner Wear Time:

Aligner wear time refers to the amount of time that each set of clear aligners should be worn by the patient each day. For effective treatment, aligners should be worn for approximately 20 to 22 hours per day, removing them only for eating, drinking, and cleaning. Consistent wear is essential for achieving the desired tooth movements and ensuring the success of the treatment.

Ortho Progress Monitoring:

Ortho progress monitoring involves regularly checking and evaluating the progress of orthodontic treatment to ensure that it is proceeding as planned. This may include periodic visits to the orthodontist for adjustments, assessments, and imaging to track tooth movement and make any necessary changes to the treatment plan. Monitoring progress helps ensure that the treatment remains on track and allows for timely interventions if issues arise.

Patient Education:

Patient education is a crucial component of orthodontic care, involving the provision of information and guidance to patients about their treatment options, the treatment process, and proper care for orthodontic appliances. Educating patients helps them understand their treatment plan, the importance of compliance, and how to maintain good oral hygiene during treatment.

Orthodontic Diagnosis and Records:

Orthodontic diagnosis and records encompass the collection and analysis of information needed to evaluate and plan orthodontic treatment. This includes diagnostic imaging, digital impressions, photographs, and clinical examinations. Accurate diagnosis and thorough records are essential for developing a personalized treatment plan and achieving optimal results.

Aligner Fit and Comfort:

Aligner fit and comfort refer to how well the clear aligners fit over the teeth and how comfortable they are for the patient to wear. Proper fit is crucial for effective tooth movement and avoiding discomfort or issues with the aligners. Patients should report any fit issues or discomfort to their orthodontist to ensure that adjustments can be made for optimal comfort and effectiveness.

Post-Treatment Care:

Post-treatment care involves the steps taken after completing active orthodontic treatment to maintain the results and ensure long-term success. This includes wearing retainers as prescribed, attending follow-up appointments, and continuing good oral hygiene practices. Post-treatment care is essential for preserving the alignment achieved and preventing teeth from shifting back.

Orthodontic Emergencies:

Orthodontic emergencies are unexpected issues or complications that may arise during orthodontic treatment, such as broken brackets, lost aligners, or severe discomfort. Patients experiencing orthodontic emergencies should contact their orthodontist promptly for guidance and resolution. Proper handling of emergencies helps minimize disruptions to the treatment process and ensures continued progress.

Orthodontic Adjustment:

Orthodontic adjustment refers to the process of making changes to orthodontic appliances, such as braces or clear aligners, to ensure that the treatment is progressing as planned. Adjustments may include changing aligners, tightening braces, or modifying the treatment plan based on the patient's progress and feedback. Regular adjustments are necessary to keep the treatment on track and achieve the desired results.

Orthodontic Retention:

Orthodontic retention is the phase of treatment where retainers are used to stabilize and maintain the results achieved with braces or clear aligners. The goal of retention is to prevent the teeth from shifting back to their original positions and ensure long-term success. Retention may involve wearing retainers full-time initially, followed by a gradual reduction in wear time as the teeth stabilize.

Clear Aligner Treatment Plan:

A clear aligner treatment plan is a detailed strategy developed by an orthodontist to guide the use of clear aligners in addressing specific dental and orthodontic issues. The plan includes information on the aligners to be used, the sequence of aligner changes, the duration of treatment, and the expected outcomes. The treatment plan is based on digital impressions, 3D modeling, and clinical assessments to ensure precise and effective results.

Orthodontic Evaluation and Diagnosis:

Orthodontic evaluation and diagnosis involve assessing a patient's dental and orthodontic condition to determine the appropriate treatment approach. This process includes a thorough examination of the teeth, jaws, and bite, as well as the use of diagnostic tools such as X-rays and digital impressions. Accurate evaluation and diagnosis are essential for developing an effective treatment plan and addressing the patient's specific needs.

Invisalign System:

The Invisalign system is a brand of clear aligners used to straighten teeth and correct orthodontic issues. Invisalign aligners are made from a flexible, medical-grade plastic material and are designed using advanced 3D technology. The system offers a range of aligner options and treatment plans tailored to address various dental concerns, from mild to moderate cases. Invisalign is known for its discreet appearance, comfort, and effectiveness.

Aligner Replacement:

Aligner replacement refers to the process of obtaining new aligners if the original set becomes damaged, lost, or needs to be adjusted. Patients should contact their orthodontist to arrange for replacement aligners and ensure that their treatment continues without interruption. Proper care and handling of aligners can help minimize the need for replacements and ensure consistent progress.

Orthodontic Treatment Goals:

Orthodontic treatment goals are the specific objectives that a patient and orthodontist aim to achieve through orthodontic therapy. These goals may include improving tooth alignment, correcting bite issues, enhancing dental aesthetics, and addressing functional concerns. Clearly defined treatment goals guide the development of a personalized treatment plan and help measure the success of the orthodontic treatment.

Patient Retention Compliance:

Patient retention compliance refers to the adherence to the retainer protocols and guidelines provided by the orthodontist after completing active treatment. Compliance with retainer wear is crucial for maintaining the alignment achieved and preventing teeth from shifting. Patients should follow the prescribed retainer schedule and attend follow-up appointments to ensure long-term treatment success.

Orthodontic Treatment Timeline:

The orthodontic treatment timeline outlines the expected duration and key milestones of orthodontic therapy. This timeline includes the phases of treatment, such as the initial consultation, active treatment with aligners or braces, and the retention phase. The timeline helps patients understand the duration of their treatment and the steps involved in achieving their orthodontic goals.

Aligner Material Science:

Aligner material science refers to the study and development of materials used in the fabrication of clear aligners. Advances in material science have led to the creation of high-quality, durable, and flexible plastics that enhance the effectiveness and comfort of aligners. Researchers and manufacturers continually explore new materials and technologies to improve aligner performance and patient satisfaction.

Orthodontic Appliance Selection:

Orthodontic appliance selection involves choosing the appropriate devices and tools for addressing a patient's specific dental and orthodontic issues. This selection is based on factors such as the severity of the issues, the patient's preferences, and the treatment goals. Options may include clear aligners, traditional braces, functional appliances, and other orthodontic devices.

Aligner Wear Schedule:

The aligner wear schedule is the recommended routine for wearing each set of clear aligners throughout the treatment process. Patients are typically instructed to wear aligners for 20 to 22 hours per day and switch to the next set of aligners according to the prescribed schedule. Adhering to the wear schedule is essential for achieving the desired tooth movements and ensuring the success of the treatment.

Orthodontic Practice Management:

Orthodontic practice management involves the administration and operation of an orthodontic practice, including aspects such as patient care, scheduling, billing, and staff management. Effective practice management ensures that the orthodontic office runs smoothly and provides high-quality care to patients. It includes implementing systems and processes for efficient treatment planning and delivery.

Orthodontic Research and Development:

Orthodontic research and development focus on advancing the field of orthodontics through innovation, experimentation, and clinical studies. This includes exploring new technologies, treatment methods, and materials to improve orthodontic care. Research and development contribute to the evolution of orthodontic practices and enhance patient outcomes.

Dental Records Management:

Dental records management involves the organization and maintenance of patient records, including diagnostic images, treatment plans, and progress notes. Accurate and up-to-date records are essential for tracking treatment progress, ensuring continuity of care, and supporting effective communication between the orthodontist and the patient.

Aligner Adjustments:

Aligner adjustments refer to modifications made to the aligner treatment plan based on the patient's progress and feedback. These adjustments may involve changing the sequence of aligners, updating the treatment plan, or addressing any issues with fit or comfort. Regular adjustments help ensure that the treatment remains effective and aligned with the patient's orthodontic goals.

Orthodontic Patient Support:

Orthodontic patient support encompasses the resources and assistance provided to patients throughout their orthodontic treatment. This includes answering questions, addressing concerns, offering guidance on aligner care and oral hygiene, and providing emotional support. Patient support is essential for ensuring a positive treatment experience and achieving successful outcomes.

FAQs about Clear Aligners

1. What are clear aligners?

    Clear aligners are removable, transparent trays used to straighten teeth gradually. They are an alternative to traditional metal braces and offer a more discreet treatment option. Unlike braces, clear aligners are made of a smooth, clear plastic material that is virtually invisible when worn.

2. How do clear aligners work?

    Clear aligners work by applying gentle, constant pressure to teeth, gradually moving them into the desired position. Each aligner in the series is custom-made based on digital impressions of your teeth and is designed to make incremental adjustments. As you progress through the series, your teeth move step-by-step toward the desired alignment.

3. How long does treatment with clear aligners take?

    Treatment duration varies depending on the complexity of the case. On average, clear aligner treatment takes between 6 to 18 months. Simple cases may require less time, while more complex cases might take longer. Your orthodontist will provide a personalized treatment timeline based on your specific needs.

4. Are clear aligners suitable for everyone?

    Clear aligners are effective for many orthodontic issues, particularly mild to moderate cases. However, they may not be suitable for complex malocclusions or severe dental issues, which may require traditional braces. Your orthodontist will evaluate your case to determine if clear aligners are the right option for you.

5. How often should I wear clear aligners?

    Clear aligners should be worn for 20 to 22 hours per day to ensure effective treatment. They can be removed for eating, drinking, and oral hygiene. Consistent wear is crucial for achieving the desired tooth movements and maintaining the treatment schedule.

6. What are the benefits of clear aligners?

    Benefits of clear aligners include improved aesthetics, comfort, and convenience. They are nearly invisible, making them a popular choice for those concerned about the appearance of metal braces. Additionally, they are removable, allowing for easier oral hygiene and fewer dietary restrictions compared to traditional braces.

7. How do I care for my clear aligners?

    Clear aligners should be cleaned regularly with a soft brush and lukewarm water. Avoid using hot water or abrasive cleaners, as they can damage the aligners. Additionally, it's important to avoid consuming staining foods and beverages while wearing the aligners to prevent discoloration.

8. What happens after treatment?

    After treatment, patients are usually required to wear retainers to maintain the results and prevent teeth from shifting back to their original positions. Retainers help stabilize the teeth in their new alignment and are typically worn full-time initially, then gradually reduced to nighttime wear.

9. Can I eat or drink with clear aligners in?

    It is recommended to remove clear aligners while eating or drinking to avoid damaging the aligners and to prevent staining. You should brush your teeth and rinse your aligners before reinserting them after meals.

10. How do I know if my clear aligners are working? Regular check-ups with your orthodontist will ensure that your treatment is progressing as planned. They will monitor the movement of your teeth and make any necessary adjustments to the treatment plan.

11. Are clear aligners more comfortable than traditional braces? Many patients find clear aligners more comfortable than traditional braces, as they do not have wires or brackets that can irritate the inside of the mouth. Clear aligners are made from smooth plastic and are custom-fitted to your teeth, minimizing discomfort.

12. Can I play sports or musical instruments with clear aligners? Yes, you can play sports or musical instruments with clear aligners. However, if you are involved in contact sports, it may be advisable to wear a mouthguard to protect your teeth and aligners. Clear aligners are removable, so you can take them out when needed and put them back in afterward.

13. Will clear aligners affect my speech? Most people experience a slight adjustment period where they may notice a slight lisp or change in speech. However, this typically resolves within a few days as you get used to speaking with the aligners in place.

14. How often will I need to visit the orthodontist during treatment? You will typically need to visit your orthodontist every 6 to 8 weeks for check-ups. These visits allow your orthodontist to monitor progress, make adjustments, and provide you with the next sets of aligners.

15. What happens if I lose or damage an aligner?

    If you lose or damage an aligner, contact your orthodontist immediately. They will provide guidance on how to proceed, which may involve wearing the previous aligner until a replacement can be made or adjustments to the treatment plan.

16. Can I switch to a different brand of aligners mid-treatment?

    Switching brands mid-treatment is not recommended, as different brands have varying technologies and treatment approaches. It is best to complete your treatment with the brand you started with to ensure consistent results.

17. Are there any restrictions on what I can eat with clear aligners?

    Unlike traditional braces, clear aligners do not have dietary restrictions, as they are removed during meals. However, you should avoid eating or drinking anything that could stain the aligners or damage them.

18. How long does it take to get used to wearing clear aligners?

    Most patients adapt to wearing clear aligners within a few days. During this time, you may experience mild discomfort or a feeling of pressure as your teeth adjust. This is normal and typically resolves as you get used to the aligners.

19. Can clear aligners fix a deep overbite or underbite?

    Clear aligners can address mild to moderate overbites and underbites. For more severe cases, traditional braces or other orthodontic treatments may be recommended to achieve the desired correction.

20. Do clear aligners require more maintenance than traditional braces?

    Clear aligners require regular cleaning and proper care to maintain their effectiveness and appearance. However, they generally require less maintenance than traditional braces, which involve more frequent adjustments and maintenance.

21. Can I use clear aligners if I have dental restorations or fillings?

    Yes, clear aligners can be used if you have dental restorations or fillings. Your orthodontist will consider these factors when planning your treatment to ensure that the aligners work effectively with your existing dental work.

22. Are clear aligners covered by dental insurance?

    Coverage for clear aligners varies by insurance plan. Some plans may cover part of the cost, while others may not. It is important to check with your insurance provider to understand your coverage and any potential out-of-pocket costs.

23. How do clear aligners compare to traditional braces in terms of effectiveness?

    Clear aligners are effective for many orthodontic issues, especially mild to moderate cases. Traditional braces may be more effective for complex cases or severe malocclusions. Your orthodontist will help determine the best option based on your specific needs.

24. Can I travel while undergoing treatment with clear aligners?

    Yes, you can travel while using clear aligners. However, it's important to ensure that you have enough aligners for the duration of your trip and to maintain your routine of wearing them as prescribed.

25. How do I know if clear aligners will work for my orthodontic issues?

    Your orthodontist will conduct a thorough evaluation, including digital scans and X-rays, to determine if clear aligners are suitable for your specific orthodontic issues. They will discuss the expected outcomes and any alternative treatment options if necessary.

26. What should I do if I experience discomfort with my clear aligners?

    Mild discomfort is normal during the initial adjustment period. If discomfort persists or becomes severe, contact your orthodontist. They can check the fit of your aligners and make any necessary adjustments to improve comfort.

27. Can clear aligners be used for children?

    Clear aligners can be used for children and adolescents, but their suitability depends on the child's dental development and specific orthodontic needs. Your orthodontist will assess whether clear aligners are appropriate or if traditional braces would be more effective.

28. What is the role of attachments in clear aligner treatment?

    Attachments are small, tooth-colored bumps bonded to your teeth to help the aligners grip and apply pressure for more complex tooth movements. They are used to enhance the effectiveness of clear aligners for specific orthodontic corrections.

29. How often should I change my clear aligners?

    You should change your clear aligners according to the schedule provided by your orthodontist, typically every 1 to 2 weeks. Changing aligners as directed is crucial for ensuring continuous progress and achieving the desired results.

30. Can I use clear aligners if I have braces on some teeth and need aligners on others?

    In some cases, a combination of braces and clear aligners may be used, depending on the complexity of the orthodontic issues. Your orthodontist will develop a treatment plan that integrates both approaches if necessary.

31. What should I do if my aligners feel too tight?

    A feeling of tightness is normal as the aligners apply pressure to move your teeth. However, if the aligners feel excessively tight or uncomfortable, consult your orthodontist. They can check the fit and make adjustments if needed.

32. Can clear aligners correct bite issues?

Yes, clear aligners can address certain bite issues, including overbites, underbites, and crossbites. However, the effectiveness depends on the severity of the bite issue. Complex bite problems may require additional treatments or traditional braces.

33. How are clear aligners different from traditional braces?

    Clear aligners are made of transparent plastic and are removable, making them less noticeable and more convenient than traditional metal braces, which are fixed to the teeth. Traditional braces consist of metal brackets and wires and may be more suitable for complex orthodontic cases.

34. Will clear aligners affect my speech?

    Some patients experience a temporary lisp or changes in their speech when they first start using clear aligners. This usually resolves within a few days as the patient adjusts to speaking with the aligners in place.

35. Can clear aligners fix gaps between teeth?

    Yes, clear aligners can effectively close gaps between teeth. The aligners gradually shift the teeth to fill the spaces, resulting in a more uniform appearance.

36. Are clear aligners less painful than traditional braces?

    Clear aligners generally cause less discomfort than traditional braces. The gradual, controlled movement of teeth with aligners usually results in less soreness and irritation compared to the frequent adjustments and pressure associated with metal braces.

37. How do I know if clear aligners are right for me?

An orthodontist will evaluate your dental and orthodontic needs to determine if clear aligners are suitable. They will consider factors like the complexity of your case, your treatment goals, and your commitment to wearing the aligners as prescribed.

38. What should I do if I lose or break an aligner?

If you lose or break an aligner, contact your orthodontist immediately. They can provide guidance on whether to proceed with the next set of aligners or order a replacement. It's important to address these issues promptly to avoid treatment delays.

39. Can I play sports with clear aligners?

Yes, you can play sports with clear aligners, but it's advisable to wear a mouthguard to protect your aligners and teeth during contact sports. Remove the aligners during the game and clean them thoroughly before reinserting them.

40. Can I smoke or use tobacco products with clear aligners?

It's best to avoid smoking or using tobacco products while wearing clear aligners, as they can stain the aligners and affect your oral health. If you do smoke, remove the aligners and clean them before reinserting them.

41. How do I handle an emergency with my aligners?

For orthodontic emergencies, such as severe discomfort or damage to the aligners, contact your orthodontist for guidance. They can advise on the next steps and schedule an appointment if needed.

42. Can I use over-the-counter whitening products with clear aligners?

It's generally not recommended to use over-the-counter whitening products while wearing clear aligners, as they can affect the aligners and may not provide even whitening. Consult your orthodontist for advice on safe whitening options.

43. What types of orthodontic issues can clear aligners address?

Clear aligners can address a range of orthodontic issues, including mild to moderate crowding, spacing, misalignment, and some bite issues. For more complex cases, traditional braces or additional treatments may be necessary.

44. How can I ensure the best results from my clear aligner treatment?

To achieve the best results, wear your clear aligners as prescribed, follow your orthodontist's instructions, maintain good oral hygiene, and attend regular check-ups. Consistent use and proper care are key to successful treatment.

45. Will my aligners be custom-made?

Yes, clear aligners are custom-made for each patient. They are created using digital impressions and 3D modeling to ensure a precise fit and effective tooth movement according to your specific treatment plan.

46. How do I know if my treatment is progressing as planned?

Your orthodontist will monitor your treatment progress through regular appointments, where they will assess the alignment of your teeth and make any necessary adjustments. You may also receive progress updates and virtual simulations to track changes.

47. What should I do if I experience discomfort with my aligners?

Some discomfort is normal as your teeth adjust to the aligners. If you experience significant pain or discomfort, contact your orthodontist. They can provide advice on managing discomfort or make adjustments if necessary.

48. Are clear aligners visible when worn?

    Clear aligners are designed to be nearly invisible, making them a discreet option for orthodontic treatment. The transparent material blends with your teeth, so they are less noticeable compared to traditional metal braces.

49. How should I store my aligners when not in use?

    Store your aligners in their designated case when not in use. This helps prevent damage, loss, or contamination. Avoid wrapping them in tissue or placing them in pockets, as they can easily be misplaced or damaged.

50. Can clear aligners be used to correct orthodontic issues in children?

Clear aligners can be used for certain orthodontic issues in children and adolescents. However, the suitability depends on the child's dental development and the complexity of the issues. Consult with an orthodontist to determine the best treatment approach for younger patients.

Additional Resources for Patients and Professionals

- **American Association of Orthodontists (AAO)**: Provides information on orthodontic treatments and finding qualified orthodontists. AAO Website

- **Invisalign**: Official website for information on Invisalign clear aligners, treatment options, and finding providers. Invisalign Website

- **ClearCorrect**: Offers details on ClearCorrect aligners, treatment plans, and provider resources. ClearCorrect Website

- **Smile Direct Club**: Provides information on direct-to-consumer aligners and treatment options. Smile Direct Club Website

- **Dental Professionals' Continuing Education**: Opportunities for dental professionals to stay updated on orthodontic advancements and clear aligner technology. CE Courses.